Key Concepts in
Nursing and
Healthcare Research

Recent volumes include:

Key Concepts in Mental Health, Second Edition

David Pilgrim

Key Concepts in Nursing

Elizabeth Mason-Whitehead, Annette McIntosh, Ann Bryan, Tom Mason

Key Concepts in Healthcare Education

Annette McIntosh, Janice Gidman, Elizabeth Mason-Whitehead

Key Concepts in Learning Disabilities

Pat Talbot, Geoff Astbury, Tom Mason

Key Concepts in Social Work Practice

Aidan Worsley, Tim Mann, Angela Olsen, Elizabeth Mason-Whitehead

Key Concepts in Public Health

Frances Wilson, Andi Mabhala

Key Concepts in Palliative Care

Moyra A. Baldwin, Jan Woodhouse

Key Concepts in Health Studies

Chris Yuill, Iain Crinson, Eilidh Duncan

Key Concepts in Anti-Discriminatory Social Work

Toying Okitikpi and Cathy Aymer

The SAGE Key Concepts series provides students with accessible and authoritative knowledge of the essential topics in a variety of disciplines. Cross-referenced throughout, the format encourages critical evaluation through understanding. Written by experienced and respected academics, the books are indispensable study aids and guides to comprehension.

Key Concepts in
Nursing and
Healthcare Research

EDITED BY ANNETTE MCINTOSH-SCOTT, TOM MASON,
ELIZABETH MASON-WHITEHEAD AND DAVID COYLE

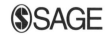

$SAGE

Los Angeles | London | New Delhi
Singapore | Washington DC

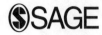

Los Angeles | London | New Delhi
Singapore | Washington DC

SAGE Publications Ltd
1 Oliver's Yard
55 City Road
London EC1Y 1SP

SAGE Publications Inc.
2455 Teller Road
Thousand Oaks, California 91320

SAGE Publications India Pvt Ltd
B 1/I 1 Mohan Cooperative Industrial Area
Mathura Road
New Delhi 110 044

SAGE Publications Asia-Pacific Pte Ltd
3 Church Street
#10-04 Samsung Hub
Singapore 049483

Editor: Alex Clabburn
Assistant editor: Emma Milman
Production editor: Thea Watson
Copyeditor: Michelle Clark
Proofreader: Bryan Campbell
Marketing manager: Tamara Navaratnam
Cover design: Wendy Scott
Typeset by: C&M Digitals (P) Ltd, Chennai, India
Printed in India by Replika Press Pvt Ltd

Library of Congress Control Number: 2013934432

British Library Cataloguing in Publication data

A catalogue record for this book is available from the British Library

ISBN 978-1-4462-1070-3
ISBN 978-1-4462-1071-0 (pbk)

DEDICATION

This book is dedicated to
Professor Tom Mason (1950–2011)

contents

contents

list of tables

list of figures

about the editors

McIntosh-Scott, Annette, PhD, BSc, Cert Ed, Dip CNE, FHEA, RGN, SCM, RNT, RCNT is Executive Dean, Faculty of Health and Social Care, University of Chester, UK.

Mason, Tom, PhD, BSc (Hons), FHEA, RMN, RNMH, RGN was Professor and Head of Mental Health and Learning Disabilities, Faculty of Health and Social Care, University of Chester, UK.

Mason-Whitehead, Elizabeth, PhD, BA (Hons), HV, PGDE, ONC, SRN, SCM is Professor of Social and Health Care, Faculty of Health and Social Care, University of Chester, UK.

Coyle, David, RN MEd RNT is a lecturer at the School of Healthcare Sciences, Bangor University, Wales, UK.

about the contributors

Alford, Simon, MSc, BSc (Hons) is a senior researcher at the Faculty of Health and Social Care, University of Chester, UK.

Aveyard, Helen, PhD, MA, BSc (Hons), PDCE, RGN is senior lecturer in Adult Nursing, School of Health and Life Sciences, Oxford Brookes University, UK.

Bryan, Ann, MSc, Cert Ed, FHEA, ADM, RGN, RM, HV, RMT is Associate Dean, Business and Enterprise, Faculty of Health and Social Care, University of Chester, UK.

Cahill, Jane, PhD, MA Hons is a senior research fellow at the School of Healthcare, University of Leeds, UK.

Deacon, Maureen, PhD, MPhil, BA Health Studies, ENB (CPN Cert), RMN, SRN is Professor of Professional Development and Head of the Department of Mental Health and Learning Disability, Faculty of Health and Social Care, University of Chester, UK.

Eost-Telling, Charlotte, PhD, MSc, BSc (Hons) is a researcher at the Faculty of Health and Social Care, University of Chester, UK.

Fallows, Stephen, PhD, BSc (Hons) is Research Coordinator, Department of Clinical Sciences, University of Chester, UK.

Flynn, Sandra, MSc, BA (Hons), RGN, ONC, DPSN is Nurse Consultant in Orthopaedics, Countess of Chester Hospital, Chester, UK.

Ford, Neville, PhD, MA, MSc, FIMA, FHEA is Executive Dean of Research, Postgraduate and Knowledge Transfer, University of Chester, UK.

Freshwater, Dawn, PhD, BA (Hons), FRCN, RN is Pro-Vice-Chancellor for Staff and Organisational Effectiveness and Professor of Mental Health, University of Leeds, UK.

Garratt, Dean, PhD, BEd (Hons), FHEA is Professor of Education, Faculty of Education and Children's Services, University of Chester, UK.

Gidman, Janice, PhD, MEd, BSc (Hons), PGCE, FHEA, ONC, RN is Head of Postgraduate Medical, Dental and Interprofessional Education and a senior teaching fellow, at the Faculty of Health and Social Care, University of Chester, UK.

Hall, Rebecca, MSc, RMN, BSc (Hons) Nursing, BSc (Hons) Community Specialist Practitioner, RMN, PGCE is a senior lecturer at the Faculty of Health and Social Care, University of Chester, UK.

Harlow, Elizabeth, PhD (social science), BA (Hons), CQSW is Professor of Social Work at the Faculty of Health and Social Care, University of Chester, UK.

Hayes, Liane, MPhil, BSc (Hons), PGCE, FHEA, MBPsS is a senior lecturer in psychology at the Faculty of Social Sciences, University of Chester, UK.

Hellenbach, Michael, PhD, MSc is a research fellow at the Faculty of Health, Life and Social Sciences, Edinburgh Napier University, Scotland, UK.

Johnson, Martin, PhD, RN is Professor in Nursing, University of Salford, UK.

Lovell, Andy, PhD, BA (Hons), Cert Ed, RNLD is Professor of Learning Disabilities at the Faculty of Health and Social Care, University of Chester, UK.

Mercer, Dave, PhD, MA, BA (Hons), PGCE, RMN is a lecturer at the School of Health Sciences, University of Liverpool, UK.

Mitchell, Andrew E.P. PhD, MSc Psychological Studies, MSc Cognitive and Behavioural Psychotherapy, BA (Hons), PGCE, RMN is a senior lecturer at the Faculty of Health and Social Care, University of Chester, UK.

Morris, Mike, PhD, MSc, BSc (Hons), FHEA is a senior lecturer at the Department of Clinical Sciences, University of Chester, UK.

Pearson, Alan, PhD, MSc, DAN, FCN, FRCN (Australia) FRCN (UK) is Professor of Evidence-Based Healthcare and Executive Director of the Joanna Briggs Institute, at the Faculty of Health Sciences, University of Adelaide, Australia.

Robertson, Debbie, PhD, BSc (Hons) Pharmacology, PGDE, RGN is a senior lecturer at the Faculty of Health and Social Care, University of Chester, UK.

Ruspini, Elisabetta, PhD is Senior Associate Professor of Sociology, at the Department of Sociology and Social Research, University of Milano-Bicocca, Italy.

Rycroft-Malone, Jo, PhD, MSc, BSc (Hons), RN is Professor of Implementation and Health Services Research, School of Healthcare Sciences, and University Director of Research, Bangor University, Wales, UK.

Sharma, Nikhil, BSc (Hons) in Medical Sciences with Management is a fourth-year medical student at King's College, London.

Sharma, Vimal Kumar, MBBS, MD, FRCPsych, PhD is Professor of International Health Development, Faculty of Health and Social Care, University of Chester,

Deputy Lead, Mental Health Research Network (NIHR) Northwest Hub and Consultant Psychiatrist, Cheshire and Wirral Partnership NHS Foundation Trust, UK.

Smith, Robin James, PhD, MSc, BSc/Econ is a lecturer at the School of Social Science, University of Cardiff, Wales, UK.

Starkey, Pat, PhD, BA (Hons) is Honorary Research Fellow, School of History, University of Liverpool, UK.

Steen, Mary, PhD, BHSc, PGCRM, PGDipHE, MCGI, ENB 997, CIMI, Counselling Cert, RGN, RM is Professor of Midwifery at the Faculty of Health and Social Care, University of Chester, UK.

Syrotiuk, Nick, MLIS, BA (Hons), BSc is a software developer for Mimas, Faculty of Humanities, University of Manchester, UK.

Thomas, Mike, PhD, MA, BNursing, Cert Ed, FHEA, RMN, RNT is Pro-Vice Chancellor (Academic) and Professor of Mental Health, University of Chester, UK.

Watson, Roger, PhD, RN, FRCN, FAAN is Professor of Nursing at the Faculty of Health and Social Care, University of Hull, UK.

Whitney-Cooper, Chris, Doctorate Professional Studies, MSc Healthcare, BSc (Hons) Nursing, SRN, RSCN, NT is Deputy Head of Acute Adult and Child Care at the Faculty of Health and Social Care, University of Chester, UK.

Wilkinson, Joyce PhD, BA (Nursing Studies), Diploma in Clinical and Pastoral Counselling, RSCN, RGN, RHV (Specialist Practitioner in Public Health Nursing) is Research Fellow at the School of Healthcare Sciences, Bangor University, Wales, UK.

Woodhouse, Jan, MEd, PGDE, BN (Hons), Dip N, RGN, OND, FETC is a senior lecturer at the Faculty of Health and Social Care, University of Chester, UK.

Worsley, Aidan, MPhil, MA Social Work (inc CQSW), BSc (Hons), Practice Teaching Award, FHEA is Professor and Dean of Social Work, University of Central Lancashire, UK.

CASE STUDY CONTRIBUTORS

Brownsell, Mike, MSc, BA (Hons), RGN, RNT, ENB 219, Dip Nursing Studies is Head of Acute Adult and Child Care in the Faculty of Health and Social Care at the University of Chester, UK.

Dulson, Julie MEd, BSc (Hons) RN Mental Health, Dip HE Nursing, ENB 998 is Faculty Co-ordinator for Pre-registration Nursing at the Faculty of Health and Social Care, University of Chester, UK.

Evers, Jean, MEd, BA (Hons) SCPHN, RN, HV is Head of Community Health and Wellbeing at the Faculty of Health and Social Care, University of Chester, UK.

Ridgway, Vicky, MA Gerontology, BSc (Hons) Nursing, PGDE, RN, ENB 998 and A34 is a senior lecturer and Project Lead at the Faculty of Health and Social Care, University of Chester, UK.

Templeman, Jenni, MRes, BCur, Dip Intensive Care Nursing Science, PGCE, RN, RM is a senior lecturer at the Faculty of Health and Social Care, University of Chester, UK.

about the contributors

introduction

An understanding of research is a fundamental requirement for any professional engaged in the delivery of healthcare practice in order to enhance the experience of service users and their carers.

It is often assumed that to engage with research requires actively writing proposals, collecting data and being involved in a highly proactive and structured way. Research activity can be embraced on many different levels, however, including reading research reports, identifying 'gaps' in the literature and in practice, presenting ideas for new research projects, disseminating findings, applying evidence to practice and evaluating the results.

Research has also been seen to be a rather enigmatic subject, full of mystery and complexities, to be engaged in by the few, not the many. Increasingly, though, research has been given more prominence in the roles of healthcare professionals, with the expectation that everyone should have the opportunity to participate in research at a level that is both appropriate and achievable for them. Research has been seen to be largely the preserve of educational institutions, but research partnerships are becoming more common, with researchers working closely with clinical colleagues, service users and carers.

As confidence with research continues to develop, so does creativity in finding new ways to understand an increasingly diverse healthcare provision. Consider for a moment how the delivery of healthcare for people with a learning disability might be enhanced. These days, having progressed from a relatively paternalistic standpoint of healthcare providers 'knowing best' to a more inclusive position of actively seeking the opinions of those who are going to use the service, the answer would be to ask them. The user's voice is now highly influential in healthcare research and those who perhaps did not have a voice in the past can be heard and help shape and improve their own care.

Research is integral to developing best practice and improving the quality of healthcare provision. Whether an individual is actively involved in doing research or in using research, an understanding of the key concepts of research is essential to be effective in any research activity.

MAKING THE MOST OF *KEY CONCEPTS IN NURSING AND HEALTHCARE RESEARCH*

This book sets out to be accessible and informative to all those engaged with research in healthcare practice or wishing to become engaged and more informed about the research process.

As with most research textbooks, it is not anticipated that *Key Concepts in Nursing and Healthcare Research* will be read in its entirety, from cover to cover. It is more likely that readers will select chapters as and when they need them.

The text is divided into four parts.

Part 1: Principles of research in healthcare provides the platform for a comprehensive understanding of enquiry and underpins the sections that follow. The place and importance of research in healthcare practice is outlined, alongside a review of the common traditions of research.

Part 2: Qualitative research methods introduces readers to the variety of methodologies that come under the umbrella of qualitative research. This section includes traditional methodologies, such as grounded theory, and less familiar ones where a creative approach is required. An example of the latter is visual research, which is as yet not well documented, but has a growing following.

Part 3: Quantitative research methods gives readers an overview of the essentials of the positivist approach to investigation in a way that is both accessible and critical.

Part 4: The research process informs readers about the research journey, from a literature review to a dissemination of findings.

Each chapter has been written by an author who has expertise in the topic covered in that chapter. The salient points of each particular concept are drawn together using the following format:

- definition
- list of key points
- discussion of the main elements of the topic
- case study, the aim of which is to illustrate and demonstrate the topic's application to healthcare practice
- conclusion
- suggestions for further reading and references.

MAKING A DIFFERENCE

Ultimately, the purpose of research activity is, in some way, to make a difference. The difference may be in the form of enhancing understanding of a particular experience or ideology. It may be to address an identified limitation in professional practice by investigating the factors involved and uncovering possible solutions. Producing robust evidence as an agent for change is fundamental to modern healthcare research. Many people reading this will be embarking on their own research studies. Such projects, particularly those at Master's level, usually involve one student pursuing a study with little or no resources at their disposal. These small projects are often thought to have only negligible impact on policy and practice, but, if they are written up as academic papers and published in the appropriate journals, they can have an impact on developing healthcare practice by, for example, being catalysts for further research.

One of the editors of this book was Professor Tom Mason (1950–2011). Tom gave an inspiring lead to many researchers and writers within the field of healthcare research, leading from the front, always encouraging and giving confidence to new generations of academic and clinical colleagues and students. He offered a characteristically simple adage, 'go on – make a difference' and we hope the readers of this book, which is Tom's last publication, will read the chapters that follow with the belief and confidence that, like Tom, they can make a difference as well.

Annette McIntosh-Scott, Elizabeth Mason-Whitehead and David Coyle
February 2013

introduction

Part 1

Principles of Research in Healthcare

1 Evidence-Based Practice and Research

Jo Rycroft-Malone

DEFINITION

The concern with providing patients with the best and safest care possible is often referred to as *evidence-based practice*. Evidence-based practice has been defined as the combination of research, clinical experience, local information and patients' preferences and experience in the delivery of care and services (Rycroft-Malone et al., 2004a). Evidence-based practice has become a policy imperative in many countries, with an associated investment in guideline development bodies, such as the National Institute for Health and Clinical Excellence (NICE, www.nice.org.uk), to support practitioners, plus services deliver on this agenda. Despite this focus and investment, there are many examples of patients receiving treatment, care and interventions that are known to be less than effective and even harmful.

There are many challenges to using evidence in practice. While practitioners genuinely wish to do the right thing for patients, robust research is just one of several components that inform health professionals in their everyday practice and many factors influence this process. The Promoting Action on Research Implementation in Health Services (PARIHS) framework provides a way of thinking about how some of these challenges can be identified and considered.

KEY POINTS

- The PARIHS framework was developed in an attempt to reflect the interdependence and interplay of the many factors that appear to play a role in the successful implementation of evidence in practice. It was developed inductively and has been refined over time (see Rycroft-Malone, 2010 and Kitson et al., 2008 for a summary)
- Successful implementation is represented as a function of the nature of *evidence*, the quality of the *context* of implementation and appropriate approaches to *facilitation*. This relationship is represented as: SI = f (E, C, F) – that is, successful implementation = function (evidence, context, facilitation)
- Evidence, context and facilitation are each positioned on a 'high' to 'low' continuum. Moving towards the high end of the continuum increases the chances

of successful implementation of evidence-based practice (Rycroft-Malone et al., 2004b)

- The proposition is that evidence-based practice is most likely to occur when evidence is scientifically robust and matches a professional consensus, patients' experiences and preferences and is informed by local information/data ('high' evidence), the context is receptive to change with appropriate cultures, leadership and robust monitoring and feedback systems ('high' context) and when there is appropriate support for change with input from skilled external and/or internal facilitators ('high' facilitation)
- The PARIHS framework should be useful for understanding some of the key ingredients of evidence-based practice, guiding evidence-based practice and as an aide-memoire in practice

DISCUSSION

See Table 1.1 for a description of the various elements and sub-elements of the PARIHS framework.

Table 1.1 Elements and sub-elements of the PARIHS framework

Elements		Sub-elements	
Evidence		**Low**	**High**
	Research	• Poorly conceived, designed and/or executed research • Seen as the only type of evidence • Not valued as evidence • Seen as certain	• Well-conceived, designed and executed research, appropriate to the research question • Seen as one part of a decision • Valued as evidence • Lack of certainty acknowledged • Social construction acknowledged • Judged as relevant • Importance weighted • Conclusions drawn
	Clinical experience	• Anecdote, with no critical reflection or judgement • Lack of consensus within similar groups • Not valued as evidence • Seen as the only type of evidence	• Clinical experience and expertise reflected on, tested by individuals and groups • Consensus within similar groups • Valued as evidence • Seen as one part of the decision • Judged as relevant • Importance weighted • Conclusions drawn
	Patient experience	• Not valued as evidence • Patients not involved • Seen as the only type of evidence	• Valued as evidence • Multiple biographies used • Partnerships with healthcare professionals • Seen as one part of a decision • Judged as relevant • Importance weighted • Conclusions drawn

Elements	Sub-elements		
Evidence		**Low**	**High**
	Local data/ information	• Not valued as evidence • Lack of systematic methods for collection and analysis • Not reflected on • No conclusions drawn	• Valued as evidence • Collected and analysed systematically and rigorously • Evaluated and reflected on • Conclusions drawn
Context		**Low**	**High**

	Culture	• Unclear values and beliefs
		• Low regard for individuals
		• Task-driven organisation
		• Lack of consistency
		• Resources not allocated
		• Not integrated with strategic goals
			• Able to define culture(s) in terms of prevailing values/beliefs
			• Values individual staff and clients
			• Promotes a learning organisation
			• Consistency of individuals' roles/ experience to value:
			  – relationships with others
			  – teamwork
			  – power and authority
			  – rewards/recognition
			• Resources – human, financial, equipment – allocated
			• Initiative fits with strategic goals and is a key practice/patient issue

	Leadership	• Traditional, command and control leadership • Lack of role clarity • Lack of teamwork • Poor organisational structures • Autocratic decisionmaking processes • Didactic approaches to learning/teaching/ managing	• Transformational leadership • Role clarity • Effective teamwork • Effective organisational structures • Democratic inclusive decisionmaking processes • Enabling/empowering approach to teaching/learning/managing

	Evaluation	• Absence of any form of feedback
		• Narrow use of performance information sources
		• Evaluations rely on single rather than multiple methods
			• Feedback on:
			  – individual
			  – team
			  – system
			  – performance
			• Use of multiple sources of information on performance
			• Use of multiple methods:
			  – clinical
			  – performance
			  – economic
			  – experience
			  – evaluations

(Continued)

Table 1.1 (Continued)

Facilitation		Low inappropriate facilitation	High appropriate facilitation
	Purpose	**Task**	**Holistic**
	Role	Doing for others:	Enabling others:
		<ul><li>episodic contact</li><li>practical/technical help</li><li>didactic, traditional approach to teaching</li><li>external agents</li><li>low intensity – extensive coverage</li></ul>	<ul><li>sustained partnership</li><li>developmental</li><li>adult learning approach to teaching</li><li>internal/external agents</li><li>high intensity – limited coverage</li></ul>
	Skills and attributes	Task/doing for others:	Holistic/enabling others:
		<ul><li>project management skills</li><li>technical skills</li><li>marketing skills</li><li>subject/technical/ clinical credibility</li></ul>	<ul><li>co-counselling</li><li>critical reflection</li><li>giving meaning</li><li>flexibility of role</li><li>realness/authenticity</li></ul>

Evidence

Within PARIHS, evidence is conceived in a broad sense to include four different types of evidence:

- research
- clinical experience
- patients' and carers' experiences
- local context information (see Rycroft-Malone et al., 2004a).

These sources of evidence are blended in decision-making to make appropriate patient-centred decisions based on the best research evidence available. This process is interactive and may need to be guided by a skilled facilitator.

Context

Context refers to the environment or setting in which the proposed change is to be implemented (see McCormack et al., 2002). The quality and nature of the contexts in which we work can have a more or less facilitative influence on our ability to change and develop practices based on evidence. Within PARIHS, the contextual factors that promote successful implementation fall under three broad sub-elements that operate in a dynamic way:

- culture
- leadership
- evaluation.

key concepts in nursing and healthcare research

6

Facilitation

Facilitation refers to the process of enabling or making easier the implementation of evidence in practice (see Harvey et al., 2002). Facilitation is achieved by an individual carrying out a specific role – that of being a facilitator, with the appropriate skills and knowledge to help individuals, teams and organisations use evidence in practice.

Facilitators have a key role to play in developing contexts that are conducive to the use of evidence. Part of this process is also about working with practitioners to help them make sense of evidence. The purpose, role, skills and attributes of facilitators are absolutely critical to implementing evidence-based practice.

CASE STUDY

PARIHS has been used in different ways (see Rycroft-Malone, 2010 for a summary). A number of tools and instruments have also been developed based on PARIHS. For example, the Context Assessment Index (McCormack et al., 2009) has been developed to assist practitioners with assessing and understanding the context in which they work and the effect this has on implementing evidence into practice. PARIHS has also been used with research and implementation activity as a conceptual and theoretical framework – that is, as an organising framework to underpin and/or guide evidence-based practice. For example, the elements can be used to understand or 'diagnose' a situation and help structure questions to make sense of situations, as follows.

Evidence

- Is there any research evidence underpinning the initiative/topic?
- Is this research judged to be well conceived, designed and conducted?
- Are the findings from research relevant to the initiative/topic?
- What is the practitioner's experience and opinion about this topic and the research evidence?
- Does the research evidence match with clinical, organisational and facilitation experience?
- Do you need to seek consensus before it might be used by practitioners in this setting? How might you do this in your workplace?
- What is the patient's experience/preference/story concerning this initiative/topic?
- Does this differ from practitioners' perspectives?
- How could a partnership approach be developed?
- Is there any robust, local information/data about the initiative/topic?

Context

- Is the context of implementation receptive to change?
- What are the beliefs and values of the organisation, team and practice context?
- What sort of leadership style is present (command and control, transformational)?

- Are individual and team boundaries clear?
- Is there effective teamworking?
- Does evaluation of performance rely on broad and varied sources of information?
- Is this information fed back to clinical contexts?

Facilitation

- Consider the answers to the evidence and context questions: what are the barriers and what are the facilitators to this initiative?
- What tasks/activities and processes require facilitation?

For a comprehensive review and critique of how PARIHS has been used previously, refer to Helfrich et al. (2010).

CONCLUSION

Evidence-based practice requires individual, team and organisational effort. Using evidence in practice is complex and challenging, which goes far beyond an individual's ability to critically appraise research. The PARIHS framework represents this complexity and provides a map of the factors that play a role and therefore need to be paid attention to in any evidence-based practice-related activities.

FURTHER READING

Rycroft-Malone, J. and Bucknall, T. (2010) *Models and Frameworks for Implementing Evidence-Based Practice*. Oxford: Wiley Blackwell.

Stetler, C.B., Damschroder, L.J., Helfrich, C.D. and Hagedorn, H.J. (2011) 'A guide for applying a revised version of the PARIHS framework for implementation', *Implementation Science*, 6: 99.

REFERENCES

Harvey, G., Loftus-Hills, A., Rycroft-Malone, J., Titchen, A., Kitson, A., McCormack, B. and Seers, K. (2002) 'Getting evidence into practice: The role and function of facilitation', *Journal of Advanced Nursing*, 37 (6): 577–88.

Helfrich, C.D., Damschroder, L.J., Hagedorn, H.J., Daggett, G.S., Sahay, A., Ritchie, M., Damush, T., Guihan, M., Ullrich, P.M. and Stetler, C.B. (2010) 'A critical synthesis of literature on the promoting action on research implementation in health services (PARIHS) framework', *Implementation Science*, 5: 82.

Kitson, A., Rycroft-Malone, J., Harvey, G., McCormack, B., Seers, K. and Titchen, A. (2008) 'Evaluating the successful implementation of evidence into practice using the PARIHS framework: Theoretical and practical challenges', *Implementation Science*, 3: 1.

McCormack, B., Kitson, A., Harvey, G., Rycroft-Malone, J., Titchen, A. and Seers, K. (2002) 'Getting evidence into practice – the meaning of "context"', *Journal of Advanced Nursing*, 38 (1): 94–104.

McCormack, B., McCarthy, G., Wright, J., Slater, P. and Coffey, A. (2009) 'Development and testing of the context assessment index (CAI)', *Worldviews on Evidence-based Nursing*, 6 (1): 27–35.

Rycroft-Malone, J. (2010) 'Promoting Action on Research Implementation in Health Services Framework', in J. Rycroft-Malone and T. Bucknall (eds), *Theory and Frameworks for Implementing Evidence-Based Practice*. Oxford: Wiley Blackwell. pp. 109–35.

Rycroft-Malone, J., Harvey, G., Seers, K., Kitson, A., McCormack, B. and Titchen, A. (2004a) 'An exploration of the factors that influence the implementation of evidence into practice', *Journal of Clinical Nursing*, 13: 913–24.

Rycroft-Malone, J., Seers, K.,Titchen, A., Harvey, G., Kitson, A. and McCormack, B. (2004b) 'What counts as evidence in evidence-based practice?', *Journal of Advanced Nursing*, 47 (1): 81–90.

2 Creating a Research-Based Culture in Healthcare Practice

Joyce Wilkinson

DEFINITION

Culture has been described as 'the way things are done around here' (Davies et al., 2000: 111). So, creating a research-based culture in healthcare practice would focus on making research a fundamental part of that, so it becomes an everyday aspect of practice. Likewise, such a culture would be one in which practice is built on research and informed by it and in which healthcare practitioners consider research when they make decisions about practice. Research-based cultures can be supported by practice development, staff development and developing research partnerships.

KEY POINTS

- Using research in practice is the cornerstone of high-quality healthcare (Parahoo, 2006) and a fundamental aspect of practice development
- Research is only one type of evidence for practice (Rycroft-Malone et al., 2004), but needs to be given consideration along with other types of information, although it may not be the first source of evidence that nurses consult (Thompson et al., 2001)
- Practice development is not only in the remit of those with specific roles but also the responsibility of all staff
- Using research in practice is broader than directly applying research findings to practice. It can also be used to improve knowledge, change attitudes and behaviour or lobby for change

- Research should form the foundation of all aspects of staff development
- Developing the capacity of individuals and teams or whole healthcare organisations to *use* research is at least as important as teaching staff about how to *do* research
- It is not necessary for all staff to have research skills as it can be embedded into policies and procedures that staff must follow, so they use research without necessarily being aware of it
- Staff development is largely an organisational responsibility, whereas practice development is often more an individual responsibility, but individuals also have to take responsibility for making the most of opportunities for staff development
- Researchers are increasingly interested in building strong partnerships with clinical staff and organisations (Rycroft-Malone, 2012). Many of these partnerships focus on doing and using research in practice, so the two are mutually important and supportive
- Research partnerships offer opportunities for staff development and practice development, providing benefits for individual staff, healthcare organisations and improving patient care

DISCUSSION

Practice development

Research and practice go hand in hand to underpin and inform the best care for patients. One without the other leads to unthinking routine and, more than ever before, there is a need to provide a sound rationale for practice (Parahoo, 2006). Research needs to be seen as one source of information on which to base decisions about the best care for patients and it can be used in the planning, provision or evaluation of changes to practice. Research can challenge or support routine practice, if the routine is subject to consideration. Taking time to think about all practice is vital (Eraut, 2004) and research can act as a stimulus and benchmark for doing so.

While there is a plethora of research about patient care, other types of research can also be useful to consider. For example, health services research considers the way in which organisations work, care is delivered or how teams work to provide care. This can also be helpful in improving or developing practice as it provides information about how to improve ways of working that can support the better delivery of care.

Practice development is not only the responsibility of those who have this in their job title but also that of all clinicians and to achieve it requires attention being given to research. It needs to be taken into consideration along with other types of evidence or knowledge, thinking through what the benefits for patients will be from its application and predicting the wider impacts of this.

Using research in practice requires thoughtful practitioners, not necessarily those who are highly skilled researchers. There are many sources of help available to support individuals and teams to become more familiar with research and start to think about how it could be used to improve patient care. Clinical nurse specialists or advanced practice nurses have expertise concerning particular clinical conditions and will also have knowledge of research relating to this. In addition, they are likely to have knowledge of doing research and how to use it in practice. Those with specific practice development roles may have responsibility for larger areas of practice, but all of these staff have core responsibilities to share their knowledge and expertise, so are a very useful starting point for using research in practice.

Using research encompasses the direct application of results to practice and a willingness to reflect on and consider practice (Janes and Fox, 2009), but can also reflect changes to attitudes and beliefs about research or can be used to lobby for change (Estabrooks, 1999; Nutley et al., 2007; Stetler, 1985). If there are not immediate opportunities to change practice, it may still be used to bring about changes over time.

Staff development

There is a clear link between developing practice and developing staff to use research to bring about improvements in care and care delivery. A research-based culture relies as much on wider staff development as it does on individuals using research as a basis for clinical care. A review of models to support evidence-based practice has shown this is a significant aspect that will determine individuals' ability to use research as much as their own skills and confidence (Wilkinson et al., 2010). Providing the organisational infrastructure to enable practitioners to use research is fundamental to ensuring that this can happen. While there would not then be an expectation that *all* clinicians would do research, there certainly should be an organisational expectation of all using research to inform practice.

While it has long been recognised that many members of staff do not have the individual knowledge and skills to use research (Estabrooks et al., 2003), there are many ways in which staff development departments can support them to do so – through the provision of research summaries or by incorporating research into organisational policies and procedures, for example. Many also provide ongoing development opportunities – such as seminars and educational programmes – and may support local initiatives for research use, such as journal clubs, or provide access to skills workshops – for example, relating to searching research databases. All depend on individuals making the most of these opportunities, acknowledging that there is need for research for practice and being proactive in accessing the necessary knowledge, skills and support, thus developing their own skills as well as the delivery of care.

Research partnerships

Research needs practice as much as practice needs research. As a result, researchers regularly seek to work with practitioners. These partnerships support a research-based culture. While research is sometimes seen as something done by a select few, there is often scope to become involved, perhaps as participants in action research projects that seek to change practice or by taking an interest in research involving patients that is taking place within organisations. There are increasing numbers of research nurses who have specific roles in research studies and who are often willing to share their knowledge and expertise, if given the opportunity to do so.

There are many opportunities for staff who would like to become more involved in research, as well as scope to develop partnerships with patients' organisations, professional organisations or local universities. Research and development departments within healthcare trusts are a good starting point as they coordinate and monitor all the research being undertaken within their organisations and can act as a source of information and contacts.

CASE STUDY

One Scottish health board provided all three means of developing a research-based culture.

Clinical nurse specialists had been involved in the development of a national research-based best practice statement for the management of continence and championed its use in their own workplace. This led to a review of practice by means of audits to consider whether or not practice reflected the recommendations for best practice, with all qualified nurses taking part in collecting audit data.

The results showed that there was considerable scope for improvements in care. At the same time, the staff development department started to provide educational sessions for healthcare assistants based on the best practice statement, as they provided much of the care relating to continence. This, in turn, fed back into practice as the healthcare assistants made simple changes to care and also felt confident enough to question decisions, such as whether or not to catheterise patients, often providing alternatives that reduced the risk of complications for patients.

The decrease in the use of catheters to manage continence led to the infection control nurse undertaking a small research study as part of her own personal professional development for a Master's degree, which involved all ward staff as partners in an action research project (Wilkinson, 2008).

CONCLUSION

This case study illustrates the different ways in which practice development, staff development and research partnerships can all contribute to the development of a research-based culture in healthcare practice that benefits all. Using research is most likely to be the way in which the majority of practitioners can influence this and, while there are both individual and organisational responsibilities involved, confidence, creativity and a willingness to reflect on practice are the most important factors for improving patient care and developing individuals' knowledge and skills. These are within the reach of every healthcare practitioner.

FURTHER READING

Wilkinson, J.E., Johnson, N. and Wimpenny, P. (2010) 'Models and approaches to inform the impacts of implementation of evidence-based practice', in D. Bick and I. Graham (eds), *Evaluating the Impact of Evidence-Based Practice*. Chichester and Oxford: Wiley-Blackwell. pp. 38–66.

REFERENCES

Davies, H., Nutley, S. and Mannion, R. (2000) 'Organisational culture and quality of healthcare', *Quality in Health Care*, 9: 111–119.

Eraut, M. (2004) 'Informal learning in the workplace', *Studies in Continuing Education*, 26 (2): 247–73.

Estabrooks, C. (1999) 'The conceptual structure of research utilization', *Research in Nursing and Health*, 22: 203–16.

Estabrooks, C., Floyd, J., Scott-Findlay, S., O'Leary, K. and Gushta, M. (2003) 'Individual determinants of research utilization: A systematic review', *Journal of Advanced Nursing*, 43 (5): 506–20.

Janes, N. and Fox, M. (2009) 'Facilitating best practice in aged care: Exploring influential factors through critical incident technique', *International Journal of Older People Nursing*, 4 (3): 166–76.

Nutley, S.M., Walter, I. and Davies, H.T.O. (2007) *Using Evidence: How research can inform public services*. Bristol: The Policy Press.

Parahoo, K. (2006) *Nursing Research. Principles, Process and Issues* (2nd edn). Houndmills, Basingstoke: Palgrave Macmillan.

Rycroft-Malone, J. (2012) 'Implementing evidence-based practice in the reality of clinical practice', *Worldviews on Evidence-based Nursing*, 9 (1): 1.

Rycroft-Malone, J., Seers, K., Titchen, A., Harvey, G., Kitson, A. and McCormack, B. (2004) 'What counts as evidence in evidence-based practice?', *Journal of Advanced Nursing*, 47 (1): 87–90.

Stetler, C.B. (1985) 'Research utilization: Defining the concept', *Image: Journal of Nursing Scholarship*, 17: 40–44.

Thompson, C., McCaughan, D., Cullum, N., Sheldon, T., Mulhall, A. and Thompson, D. (2001) 'Research information in nurses' clinical decision making: What is useful?', *Journal of Advanced Nursing*, 36 (3): 376–88.

Wilkinson, J.E. (2008) 'Managing to implement evidence-based practice?: An exploration and explanation of the roles of nurse managers in supporting evidence-based practice implementation'. PhD thesis, University of St Andrews.

Wilkinson, J.E., Johnson, N. and Wimpenny, P. (2010) 'Models and approaches to inform the impacts of implementation of evidence-based practice', in D. Bick and I. Graham (eds), *Evaluating the Impact of Evidence-Based Practice*. Chichester and Oxford: Wiley-Blackwell. pp. 38–66.

3 The Research Journey

Rebecca Hall and Elizabeth Mason-Whitehead

DEFINITION

The research journey – irrespective of the complexities or size of the study – follows a pattern of stages that is often known as the 'research process' and provides a recognised framework for the project planning, design and presentation of results. The starting point of the research journey is having a common understanding and definition of the term 'research', as described by Parahoo (2006: 472):

> It is the study of phenomena by rigorous and systematic collection and analysis of data. It is a private enterprise made public for the purposes of exposing it to scrutiny of others, to allow for replication, verification or falsification.

Where possible in this chapter we also discuss the personal research journey and we ask you to consider at what stage you see yourself in this process. Importantly, research is a continuing learning trajectory whatever your level of expertise or experience.

KEY POINTS

- The research process is a timely and scientific enquiry, with the intention of generating new knowledge
- Those involved in healthcare need to develop an awareness of the research that underpins practice. It improves the care given and enhances the experience of receiving care
- Healthcare research deepens our understanding of the concepts central to the profession. It does not need to be complicated in order to develop new insights into nursing practice
- The outcome of blending the best available research and expert clinical opinion, in addition to recognising patient preference, is called evidence-based practice

DISCUSSION

In this section we suggest that the 'research journey' consists of two journeys. The first is about your personal research journey and the second relates to the journey of the research process itself.

Your personal research journey

This is a journey of continued learning, building personal confidence, experience and expertise within the discipline of research. Take a few moments to look at Figure 3.1 and, using the following notes, consider which stage of the personal journey pyramid most closely fits your experience and expertise.

- **Research awareness** This is the experience of people who are just being introduced to research and beginning to have an awareness of its presence and significance in our everyday and professional lives. They may have an outline understanding of the complexities and breadth of research and may have been introduced to some fundamental terms, such as 'quantitative' and 'qualitative'.
- **Research familiarity** is experienced by people who have developed their awareness into something more tangible and perhaps taken steps to understand something of research, such as reading textbooks and academic journals.
- **Research engagement** This suggests a real commitment to wanting to go beyond familiarisation with research and become as knowledgeable as possible about

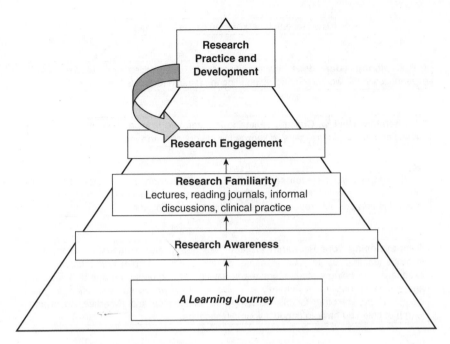

Figure 3.1   Personal research journey pyramid

methodologies, designs and applications. People with such engagement will take opportunities to attend research lectures and conferences and read as widely as possible, with a view to getting more involved, in a 'hands on' manner, in a research study, perhaps in the role of a research assistant or participating in bid writing.

- **Research practice and development** involves people who have been through the previous stages and found engagement with research to be an exciting and rewarding endeavour. At this point, researchers may be writing bids and looking critically to see opportunities where research findings may, for example, develop professional practice.

The research journey

Undertaking your first research study can, not surprisingly, be a daunting prospect. Students often approach their first study with a 'hunch' that an area of practice they have been engaged in is not delivering the best care. Their proposed research will identify the problem and hope to provide evidence that will be an agent for change. The proposed projects can be too ambitious and students usually need to be reminded that they are one person carrying out one piece of research with non-existent funds!

The aim of Figure 3.2 is to give students confidence and provide order for their research, facilitating both new and more experienced researchers by providing an anchor and plan for what may be a long journey.

There are many ideas and concepts to be mindful of when embarking on any research journey and you may wish to begin by challenging some of your own thoughts. For example, as a health practitioner, how do you see your role as a

The Research Journey: 10 Steps to Success

1 – **Exploring your Ideas.** Having discussions with colleagues, utilising your experiences in the workplace and responding to research requests from your employer.

2 – **Literature Review.** Critically reviewing the literature to gain a command of your subject and ascertain the 'gaps' in knowledge in your chosen area.

3 – **Developing your Research Question.** Your line of inquiry will depend upon a number of factors including amalgamating your ideas as well as contributing to existing knowledge and possible research questions from your employer.

4 – **Developing your Research Project.** Your design and methods will in the first instance depend upon your research question. For example 'understanding the experiences of being a student nurse and having children under the age of 3 years of age' suggests that this is primarily a qualitative study, which you will reflect in your design. There are other factors including your experience and expertise, costs and length of time you have to conduct your investigation.

5 – **Designing your Research Proposal.** The half-way stage of your journey brings together a coherent proposal that can be implemented by another researcher as well as yourself. It is important that every stage of the research proposal is fully explained and all the necessary and relevant information should be included.

6 – **Ethical Approval.** Being an ethical researcher is a fundamental pre-requisite to health care research. The ethical approval process can be daunting but taking time to understand the process from the beginning of your study will help ensure you are prepared for your application to the Ethics Committee.

7 – **Data Collection.** Preparing your field work in advance will ensure that this is one of the most enjoyable steps on your research journey. It is your only opportunity to engage with your participants and feel confident that at last you are a researcher!

8 – **Analysis and Interpretation.** With careful planning of your analysis of data using a recognised research design and theoretical framework, you will soon see how your research unfolds to reveal anticipated and unexpected findings.

9 – **Dissemination of Findings.** This important step of the journey involves conveying your findings to a relevant and interested audience through for example; reports, conference presentations, seminars and journal publications.

10 – **Application of Findings to Practice.** Your findings may directly develop practice but equally they may act as a catalyst for further research which ultimately becomes the agent for change.

Figure 3.2 The research journey

researcher and does it complement or compromise your profession? Do you see a place for traditional practice that is not based on research but on customs that have been passed down through generations of members of your profession?

It is not uncommon for people to feel anxious about embarking on this journey, because they feel they do not have the knowledge that is required to conduct research. Yet, as Figure 3.1 indicates, we are all at different stages and all of us are learning. Usually, there is ample support for your research study and you should be guided by your supervisors or academic tutors. It is important that you know where to seek advice and that your voice is being heard.

Gomm (2008: 20, 21) reminds us that 'research is about producing knowledge' and discusses the importance of being objective, advising that it is 'relatively easy for quantitative researchers to give an objective account'. To help the researcher establish whether or not the research knowledge is objective, Gomm (2008) has identified a number of criteria to use as a guide, including:

- the assumptions made about the nature of reality
- the questions asked
- the methods used for data collection
- the findings
- the answer given to the research question
- the presentation of findings that are open to scrutiny.

The research journey is one of producing knowledge through accountability, integrity, honesty and learning.

CASE STUDY

Angus was a third-year student nurse and, despite achieving good results during years one and two, he had concerns about the research module. Working as a healthcare assistant during his gap year had prepared him well for the programme – mentors reported that he settled into placement areas with ease and he was seen to be keen and quick to learn. In class, he contributed to discussions and was regarded as a confident, competent, student. He fully understood the need for an evidence base in nursing, but identifying a research focus for Angus' dissertation was proving to be a challenge. Research language seemed difficult for him to understand and his ideas seemed too broad or complicated.

While on placement, an invitation was circulated encouraging interested staff to attend a research event. The day would provide an insight into research activity within the trust. Angus had discussed his concerns with his mentor and she felt that this would be a good opportunity to develop ideas and dispel concerns.

Angus went and listened to the presentations and considered the posters people had displayed. He was amazed at the diversity of the research taking place and how much he was able to understand in terms of the research process. To hear the rationale for these studies and observe the various methodologies used was inspiring. Angus was surprised at the simple, yet logical approach that some researchers adopted. He also felt encouraged that those conducting research were mostly healthcare professionals. He started to think about what, in his experience, could improve or enhance patients' experiences of services, no matter how small. Angus realised that research does not have to be complicated. Once he had identified an area of interest to be investigated, the research 'language' that had caused him anxiety began to make sense.

CONCLUSION

In this chapter we suggested that the research journey, often known as the research process, is entwined with your personal research journey. Your research project develops simultaneously with your own development, confidence and expertise. These journeys unite a range of professional skills and personal emotions and the outcome will hopefully be a rewarding experience and an indication that a contribution, however small, to the existing body of knowledge has been made.

FURTHER READING

Bowling, A. (2009) *Research Methods in Health* (3rd edn). Maidenhead: Open University Press.
Rallis, S.F. and Rossman, G. (2012) *The Research Journey: Introduction to inquiry*. New York: Guilford Press.
Roberts, C.M. (2010) *The Dissertation Journey: A practical and comprehensive guide to planning, writing and defending your dissertation*. London: Sage.

REFERENCES

Gomm, R. (2008) *Social Research Methodology. A critical introduction* (2nd edn). Houndmills, Basingstoke: Palgrave Macmillan.
Parahoo, K. (2006) *Nursing Research Principles, Process and Issues* (2nd edn). Houndmills, Basingstoke: Palgrave Macmillan.

4 Paradigms and Philosophies

Mike Thomas

DEFINITION

'Epistemology', in philosophy, is the theory of knowledge, especially the analysis of its methods, validity and scope. It concerns itself with both the acquisition and limits of human knowledge and explores elements of science, such as evidence and methods of enquiry, as well as cognitive processes that make sense of knowledge, such as perception, sensory input, memory, beliefs and cultural contexts.

Knowledge is generally held to be based on three points Plato set out in his writings:

- a person has knowledge if there is a belief in the knowledge (for example, I am hungry)
- the knowledge is true (I have not eaten for several hours)
- there are good grounds for having belief in the truthfulness of the knowledge, it can be justified (this experience has occurred before).

This approach is open to challenge and many philosophers have grappled with variations on knowledge and truth. Russell (1967) argued that there are different types of knowledge and, while some may be based on personal beliefs (internalised knowledge of sensory input, for example), some are proposed to us by others (propositional knowledge) and, therefore, require different perceptions of trust and evidence. Another view is that knowing *about* something is different from knowing *how* to do something.

In the late seventeenth century, Locke (1961) took an empiricist view that knowledge is derived from a mental perception of the senses and experiences. Rationalists such as Descartes (Cottingham, 1997) counter-proposed that knowledge based on perception may be erroneous and argued that a heightened sense of reason and rationality is needed to demonstrate the evidence-base of knowledge. This debate continues to the present day as new technology, techniques and methods of inquiry suggest that many suppositions and assumptions underpinning what we know are erroneous. This means that epistemology, of necessity, seeks to understand the concept of truth and the beliefs out of which the emphasis on scientific methodologies has grown and the consequential quest for reliability, validity, repeatability and the ability to generalise.

Such a rationalist and sceptical approach provides the basis for scientific paradigms and is the drive behind wanting to find the 'theory of everything', but it is not without its detractors. The phenomenological approach to science suggests that we can never truly know everything and all we have is a contextual truth, based on the time and place of existence.

The term 'paradigm' was popularised by Kuhn's (1970) work on scientific structures when he used it to describe types of thinking specific to particular assumptions and approaches used in different research methods. It is applied to the research approaches used by different schools to explore phenomena. For example, researchers appear to prefer positivist, naturalistic or constructivist paradigms, each with their own rules and expectations with regard to research activities. Paradigmatic thinking helped science to understand that there are different methodical approaches to scientific endeavours that support epistemology.

KEY POINTS

- Epistemology is the study of knowledge itself – how it is structured and demonstrated and how beliefs and cognitive processes work to support trust in knowledge
- Paradigms are different approaches to scientific inquiry each with their own beliefs, assumptions and methodical techniques

Epistemology is often confused and used interchangeably with ontology, but they are different branches of the philosophy of knowledge. 'Ontology' can be summarised as the study of the *characteristics* of reality, or being, while epistemology studies *how* we know about reality (Gomm, 2004). To make matters worse, some branches of existential and phenomenological philosophy use the term ontology to refer to the study of essence or existence.

Irrespective of philosophical concerns, what is important is to have a 'purpose', sometimes referred to as a 'justification', for a study (Clough and Nutbrown, 2007); in other words, is the phenomenon to be studied real? If so, then there will be assumptions made about the researcher's own approach. For example, if a researcher wishes to study nursing in the community, there are three options for how this can be done:

- by going out with district nurses and working alongside them – a 'naturalistic' approach
- by measuring pre- and post-intervention scores and outcomes data – a 'positivist/ empirical' approach
- by exploring nursing via the experiences and thoughts of the district nurses – a 'phenomenological' approach.

Researchers have their own views about which is the best approach, often based on their assumptions, beliefs and knowledge about the area to be studied. They may believe that there needs to be strict control of the variables to be measured and the potential for intervention and influence on the experimental process need to be minimised. Alternatively, they may believe that reality is a social or personal construct, a subjective experience and only by interacting with the subjects themselves can patterns emerge.

Understanding your own paradigm approach is an important first step in research design as beliefs and assumptions about gathering data will determine which research method will be appropriate. The main two categories are 'quantitative' and 'qualitative'. These each have various methodological approaches that can be used, such as, for quantitative methods, deduction, experimental design and statistical analysis, and, in qualitative methods, induction, interpretation and flexible designs.

The terms 'positivism' and 'empiricism' are used to describe a scientific approach that rejects ideas not necessarily based on fact in favour of a pragmatic approach using valid measurements to collect evidence. It is the most dominant paradigm in the field of scientific inquiry because of its emphasis on description, explanation and empirical facts.

Originally, positivism/empiricism was accepted as an approach that was applicable in both the physical *and* social sciences, but the growth of the logical positivism movement (also known as logical empiricism) in the mid-twentieth century, with its stress on rationality using mathematical analysis, means that, today, it is almost exclusively used to describe quantitative empirical approaches. It is still used in economics and public health where there is an emphasis on epidemiology and statistical analysis.

Interestingly, 'post-positivism' somewhat undermines the positivists' assumption by using qualitative in addition to quantitative analysis, to double-check the results of experiments (Blaxter et al., 2006). Post-positivists believe that research gives only a partial glimpse of reality, but, nevertheless, they prefer the more detached, mathematical assumptions of positivism, with qualitative methodologies used as comparators for numerical results rather than being the primary methodology.

'Naturalistic' paradigms have some links with positivism, but assume that our reality is only a part of nature, time and space. The preferred approach is to study phenomena in a natural setting. Naturalism begins to separate from the positivist paradigm in its acceptance that some areas of study may initially appear to be outside mathematical formulae (for example, societal culture or attitudes), but they are still rational as every study gives a *glimpse* of reality, never the full picture.

This assumption can be confused with 'phenomenology' as some use the term to denote naturalistic approaches (Polit et al., 2001). It differs from the phenomenological method of the same name, however, which studies how individuals make sense of their own reality via individual experiences.

Naturalistic paradigms gather evidence to produce theory that can later be tested as technologies and techniques develop and are primarily used in the fields of psychology, sociology, biological and environmental sciences.

'Constructive' or 'interpretative' paradigms reject the positivist assumption of there being one objective reality that can be measured. Constructivism is an approach that accepts knowledge as not something acquired as if from nowhere, but a product of effort and cognitive processing. Constructivists understand reality via the assumptions we make that build on existing knowledge, which may be erroneous or eventually become extinct. Different observers invent their own explanations about the same phenomena and it is their scientific inquiry into these that produces tools to support their theories. Methodologies are invented to reinforce existing knowledge rather than discover completely new knowledge, as knowledge is constantly based on previous studies and findings.

The constructivist paradigm can be observed when researchers defend theories that cannot yet be tested or demonstrated via traditional positivist or naturalist approaches. Constructivists, therefore, reject metaphysical ideas but do accept that reality is socially constructed and there are as many realities as there are people to interpret them (Robson, 2011). Constructivism/interpretivism can be seen in research carried out in areas such as quantum physics, economics, psychology, learning theory and theory construction.

CASE STUDY

Elisabeth is a nurse who is undertaking a Masters degree at a local university. She has to choose a project for her research dissertation and wants to study what patients think about the care given on her ward.

Elisabeth was perfectly clear about her study topic until she started to read around research and all the different terms and definitions, often used interchangeably, and became confused about her research approach. She went to see her supervisor, who suggested they started from the beginning and asked why

Elisabeth wanted to carry out her study – whether it was for policy purposes, quality purposes or to involve patients in the operational aspects of care? Elisabeth decided that she wanted to find out if the patients liked the care and so her study would be centred on quality issues.

With her supervisor, Elisabeth began to explore what type of evidence would answer her question: what do patients think about the care given on the ward? There was currently a focus on care, compassion and patient dignity, so Elisabeth knew she could get existing questionnaires and interview schedules. Her supervisor then asked Elisabeth to explain in detail what she wanted to explore: was it a focus on causative factors, identifying areas that cause positive or negative reactions (noises at night, for example), or was her study trying to find out what could be done to improve future care? Elisabeth decided on the latter and went on to discuss the ethical and organisational regulations to be addressed before her study could commence (Mason, 2002). The session ended with a summary of the above stages and contextualising them within an epistemological framework.

Elisabeth left the supervisory session much clearer about the approach for her dissertation. In epistemological terms, she was taking a constructivist/interpretative paradigm because she was interested in, and believed (assumed), that the patients made sense of their own realities and would have different perceptions of their care. Elisabeth believed strongly in the individualisation of care, so this paradigm fitted in with her worldview and beliefs.

Within her interpretative paradigm she planned to use a qualitative method and utilise both questionnaires and focus group interviews to gather data. These are validated tools, used with existing measuring instruments (questionnaire/interviews), so would give her study both reliability and validity and allow her to plan and implement an enhanced patient care programme.

CONCLUSION

Although it is not imperative that healthcare staff become deeply immersed in philosophical discussions about the nature of reality and existence (ontology) or how we know what we know (epistemology), an understanding of how knowledge is gained and the methods for gaining that knowledge (paradigms) is important in clinical care. By understanding the pre-study assumptions and beliefs about scientific approaches made by researchers, the reader of a published study is better able to critique the method, data collection, analysis and conclusions and judge whether the findings are relevant to their care environment or not. It also allows for a higher level of understanding regarding the reliability and validity of the findings.

Equally important, by exploring their own beliefs and assumptions about how knowledge is gained, healthcare professionals can develop an understanding of research paradigms, methods and the methodologies regarding their topics of study that they could use and best suit their worldviews.

FURTHER READING

Clough, P. and Nutbrown, C. (2007) *A Student's Guide to Methodology* (2nd edn). London: Sage.
Robson, C. (2011) *Real World Research* (3rd edn). Oxford: Wiley-Blackwell.

REFERENCES

Blaxter, L., Hughes, C. and Tight, M. (2006) *How to Research* (3rd edn). Maidenhead: Open University Press.

Clough, P. and Nutbrown, C. (2007) *A Student's Guide to Methodology* (2nd edn). London: Sage.

Cottingham, J. (1997) *Descartes.* London: Orion.

Gomm, R. (2004) *Social Research Methodology; A critical introduction.* Houndmills, Basingstoke: Palgrave Macmillan.

Kuhn, T.S. (1970) *The Structure of Scientific Revolutions* (2nd edn). Chicago, IL: University of Chicago Press.

Locke, J. (1961) *An Essay Concerning Human Understanding.* New York: Dutton.

Mason, J. (2002) *Qualitative Researching.* London: Sage.

Polit, D.F., Beck, C.T. and Hungler, B.P. (2001) *Essentials of Nursing Research: Methods, appraisals and utilization* (5th edn). New York: Lippincott.

Robson, C. (2011) *Real World Research* (3rd edn). Oxford: Wiley-Blackwell.

Russell, B. (1967) *The Problems of Philosophy.* Oxford: Oxford University Press.

5 Qualitative Research

Ann Bryan with case study by Vicky Ridgway

DEFINITION

'Qualitative research' is a systematic and subjective approach that is used to find out more about the ways in which people interact and make sense of their experiences of the world. It is derived from the humanistic disciplines of social anthropology and sociology, where the purpose is to understand or interpret people's behaviour and explain the dynamics of society. Whereas quantitative methodologies test theory deductively from existing knowledge, qualitative researchers are guided by various ideas, perceptions or hunches regarding the subject of the investigation (Gerrish and Lacey, 2010). Thus, they develop theory inductively. According to Burns and Grove (2009), qualitative research contains many realities that are constantly changing and meaning is set in a given context or situation.

KEY POINTS

- Qualitative research has an important role to play in the delivery of healthcare. It can help health professionals to make sense of individuals' experiences and use the acquired knowledge to improve the quality of care
- An appropriate framework is essential for a sound, systematic and structured qualitative research approach

DISCUSSION

Qualitative research helps us to understand human experiences. It has a person-centred and holistic perspective, which is obviously important for healthcare professionals, who are involved in direct patient contact. The knowledge generated by qualitative research informs the basis of decisions that affect health and well-being. Qualitative approaches are extremely useful for examining areas where there is a lack of knowledge. They can make sense of multifaceted situations and give new insights into phenomena (Richards and Morse, 2007). Furthermore, qualitative research is suitable for investigating the complexities of the social, economic, political and environmental factors that need to be focused on by health professionals.

There is a wide range of qualitative research methodologies and methods, but, as Holloway and Wheeler (2009) state, they all have a number of characteristics and procedures in common:

- qualitative research takes the 'emic' perspective, which means the understanding that human behaviour can only be understood from the insider's point of view
- the researchers immerse themselves in the environment and culture that is being investigated
- there is a close relationship between the researcher and the participants involving mutual trust and respect.

Research frameworks

When undertaking qualitative research, one of the major challenges is understanding the language involved in the process. The terminology is far from consistent and is often used interchangeably (Welford et al., 2011). It is possible to avoid some of the confusion and ambiguity, however, by using a reliable framework to consider the various elements that constitute this approach.

It is a prerequisite that all qualitative researchers have an underpinning paradigm that fits the research to be undertaken. 'Paradigms' are sets of ideas about the phenomena under investigation. According to Crotty (1998), they are characterised by the following four basic elements that inform each other.

- **Methods** The procedures or techniques used to gather and analyse data related to a research question.
- **Methodology** The strategy, plan of action or design behind the choice of particular methods that links the choice of methods to the desired outcomes.
- **Theoretical perspective** The philosophical stance informing the methodology, providing a context for the process and grounding its logic and criteria.
- **Epistemology** The theory of knowledge embedded in the theoretical perspective and thereby in the methodology. A way of understanding and explaining how we know what we know.

Crotty (1998) further postulates that, using this framework, we can effectively analyse and understand the qualitative research process, although he acknowledges that no one paradigm is superior to another. As Weaver and Olsen (2006) argue, different paradigms can make valuable contributions to different areas of health-care practice. Furthermore, the elements of the research framework cannot be considered in isolation because they have a fundamental impact on each other.

Methods

Qualitative research is characterised by using methods that are interpretative and centre on meaning (Richards and Morse, 2007). There is a wide range of these methods available for data collection and analytical strategies – Tesch (1990) maintains their number exceeds 40. It is a challenge, therefore, for researchers to choose one that is appropriate in relation to meeting the aims of the study, but the most commonly used methods include structured and semi-structured interviews, participant and non-participant observation and document analysis. The principle objective is to understand the meaning and significance of lived experiences, which, in turn, generate in-depth descriptions of phenomena.

Methodology

Methodology is connected with the process and procedure for acquiring know-ledge. It influences the choice and use of particular methods and links them to a study's aims (Crotty, 1998). Only when the methodology is decided should researchers consider which methods should be used to collect and analyse data. The underlying strength of qualitative research methodologies is that they have an holistic approach that is flexible.

There are several qualitative methodologies of choice for healthcare research. Those most frequently employed can be summarised as follows.

- **Ethnography** This is the oldest of all the qualitative methodologies. Ethnographers focus on cultures and involve themselves in the collection, description and analysis of data to develop a theory of cultural behaviour.
- **Phenomenological research** A strategy of enquiry that emphasises the complexity of human experience and the need to study that experience holistically as it is actually lived.
- **Grounded theory** A research methodology that uses inductive and deductive approaches to generate theory from the data by means of constant comparison.
- **Action research** An interactive enquiry process concerned with developing practical knowledge to enable the realisation of worthwhile human purposes. It aims to 'bring together action and reflection, theory and practice, in participation with others, in the pursuit of practical solutions to issues of pressing concern to people' (Reason and Bradbury, 2008: 1).
- **Mixed methods** A research technique that combines alternative approaches in a single research project. It recognises that individual methodologies have limitations and by mixing methods these limitations can be overcome.

Theoretical perspective

Traditionalists maintain that it is necessary for the researcher to have an understanding of the philosophical ideas on which the choice of methodology and method are based (Reeves et al., 2008). This understanding is embedded in the assumptions brought to the research task. 'Assumptions' are basic principles that are accepted as being true on the basis of logic or reason, without proof or verification (Polit and Beck, 2008), and are reflected in the methodology. It is essential to consider these assumptions and explain them. This can be achieved by developing a theoretical perspective that, according to Crotty (1998: 7) is 'our view of the human world and social life within that world, wherein such assumptions are grounded'.

The most frequently adopted theoretical perspectives in qualitative healthcare research include interpretative research, critical theory, feminism and pragmatism. 'Interpretative research' has a long history dating back to the late nineteenth century. It aims to make sense of and find meaning in human experience from different perspectives (Weaver and Olsen, 2006), including symbolic interactionism and the various branches of phenomenology.

'Critical theory' and 'feminism' are often discussed together as both theoretical perspectives maintain that certain groups suffer because of the way power is structured throughout society. Traditionally, critical theorists claim that it is the working classes who are disadvantaged, whereas the feminist standpoint is that women are disadvantaged.

'Pragmatism' is concerned with determining the value of an idea by its outcome in practice (Weaver and Olsen, 2006). Claims to knowledge develop from actions, situations and consequences. The pragmatic approach enables healthcare professionals to progress beyond the boundaries of a single theoretical perspective towards the construction of theories that are adapted to fit particular situations (Doane, 2003).

Epistemology

Whereas the theoretical perspective is how we view the world and understand it, 'epistemology' is the theory of knowledge itself, concerned with the ways in which human beings know the world (Holloway and Wheeler, 2009). It is inherent in the theoretical perspective and, therefore, in the methodology selected (Crotty, 1998). There are three main epistemological stances:

- objectivism
- constructionism
- subjectivism.

'Objectivists' believe that researchers can observe the world objectively without contaminating a study. 'Constructionists' claim that human beings make sense of their experience by constructing meaning, so it is not possible for a researcher to maintain a detached objective observer. In 'subjectivism', meaning is not established via an interaction between subject and object, but is forced on the object by the subject.

A further branch of philosophy that needs to be considered alongside epistemology is 'ontology'. According to Denzin and Lincoln (1994), ontology questions what is the real world and what can be known about it. This is different from epistemology, which questions the relationship between the knower and what can be known. In practice, however, ontological and epistemological issues have a tendency to materialise at the same time. Hence, it is necessary for the two perspectives to be consistent so that researchers are able to generate sound knowledge and explanations about the world in which we live and interact.

CASE STUDY – VICKY RIDGWAY

The following case study outlines a qualitative research approach, from the underpinning epistemology, theoretical perspective and methodology to the method used to collect the data.

Sally, a nurse caring for older people, decided, as part of her postgraduate studies that she would like to examine clients' transition from acute hospital care to long-term care. She had previously observed, in clinical practice, that clients and their families became anxious during this process. Having completed an initial review of the literature, however, she could find no evidence to support her observations. She decided to use the semi-structured interview method with older people to establish how they coped with the transition to long-term care. This method was based on her choice of grounded theory methodology, which would allow her to gather and analyse data with the aim of developing theories grounded in real-world observations.

Sally chose this particular methodology because the theoretical perspective underpinning grounded theory is symbolic interactionism, which focuses on the interactions between people as a means of exploring human behaviour. The epistemology inherent in symbolic interactionism and also in the chosen methodology is constructionism. She found this appropriate because constructionists consider that meaning is only extracted when a person engages in an activity and meaning can then be discovered.

The strength of Sally's research design gave her the foundation she needed to take her proposal forward. The philosophical underpinning embedded in constructionism and symbolic intractionism, together with the methodology of grounded theory and the method of semi-structured interviews, created an appropriate framework for a sound, systematic and structured qualitative research study.

CONCLUSION

The practice of basing qualitative research in paradigms, together with the subsequent knowledge resulting from the research process, can only be of value if it enhances healthcare delivery and individual well-being. Hence, it is necessary to use a reliable framework that makes it possible to effectively analyse and understand the various elements that constitute the qualitative approach. For example, Crotty's (1998) framework enables the researcher to choose the method, methodology, theoretical perspective, epistemology and ontology that best fit the requirements of the proposed research study.

Crotty, M. (1998) *The Foundations of Social Research: Meaning and perspective in the research process.* London: Sage.

REFERENCES

Burns, N. and Grove, S.K. (2009) *The Practice of Nursing Research: Appraisal, synthesis and generation of evidence* (6th edn). St Louis, MO: Saunders Elsevier.

Crotty, M. (1998) *The Foundations of Social Research: Meaning and perspective in the research process.* London: Sage.

Denzin, N.K. and Lincoln Y.S. (1994) *Handbook of Qualitative Research.* London: Sage.

Doane, G.H. (2003) 'Through pragmatic eyes: Philosophy and the re-sourcing of family nursing', *Nursing Philosophy,* 4 (1): 25–32.

Gerrish, K. and Lacey, A. (2010) *The Research Process in Nursing.* Oxford: Wiley-Blackwell.

Holloway, I. and Wheeler, S. (2009) *Qualitative Research in Nursing and Healthcare* (3rd edn). Oxford: Wiley-Blackwell.

Polit, D.F. and Beck, C.T. (2008) *Nursing Research: Generating and assessing evidence for nursing practice.* Philadelphia, PA: Lippincott.

Reason, P. and Bradbury, H. (2008) *Handbook of Action Research: Participative inquiry.* London: Sage.

Reeves, S., Albert, M., Kuper, A. and Hodges, B.D. (2008) 'Why use theories in qualitative research?', *British Medical Journal,* 337: 949.

Richards, L. and Morse, J.M. (2007) *Read Me First for a User's Guide to Qualitative Methods* (2nd edn). London: Sage.

Tesch, R. (1990) *Qualitative Research: Analysis types and software tools.* London: Falmer.

Weaver, K. and Olsen, J.K. (2006) 'Understanding paradigms used for nursing research', *Journal of Advanced Nursing,* 53 (4): 459–69.

Welford, C., Murphy, K. and Casey, D. (2011) 'Demystifying nursing research terminology: Part 1', *Nurse Researcher,* 18 (4): 38–43.

key concepts in nursing and healthcare research

28

6 Quantitative Research

Charlotte Eost-Telling

DEFINITION

'Quantitative research' methods are used to measure the quantity or number of a characteristic or characteristics. Empirical evaluations are utilised and the results analysed using mathematical and statistical analysis. The aim of quantitative research is to determine the relationship between one or more characteristics (the independent variables) and another or others (the dependent variables) in a population. This is achieved by developing and applying mathematical models, theories or hypotheses to phenomena in an organised, systematic way, enabling the findings to be generalised to other situations or populations being studied. Measurement is central to quantitative research because it provides the fundamental connection between empirical observation and mathematical expression of relationships.

KEY POINTS

- Quantitative research is essential to the development of evidence-based practice. It can be used to describe, explain, predict and control phenomena in healthcare
- It is important to approach quantitative research in a systematic, structured and objective way, to minimise the effect of both human bias and extraneous variables
- The use of controls, predetermined research instruments and statistical analyses contribute to the accuracy of the research data in reflecting reality and enable a study's findings to be generalised to the whole of the population being studied

DISCUSSION

Epistemology and ontology

Quantitative research has its origins in the physical sciences, the modern philosophy of quantitative research emerging from Comte's positivist framework (Bruce et al., 2008; Creswell, 2008). Researchers espousing this philosophy believe that the aim of knowledge is to describe phenomena which are experienced and that there is 'one' definitive answer to a research question waiting to be discovered via observation and measurement. This truth allows us to predict and control further variables in the future.

Positivists, including logical positivists, consider, that since emotions cannot be seen, they cannot be measured, and only phenomena fully explainable scientifically can be used to advance science. More recently, however, some researchers have moved beyond positivism to a post-positivist perspective (Trochim, 2006). This approach theorises that, although there is indeed a universal truth which can be measured, we have not yet fully discovered it. Direct observation and measurement help move us towards the truth, but there are still unknown elements as yet to be researched and understood.

Other schools of thought believe that qualitative and quantitative research methods should not be seen as dichotomous, but as a spectrum accommodating both fields of research (Creswell and Plano Clark, 2007). This acknowledges that most research is a combination of both quantitative and qualitative methods and that much quantitative research is based on qualitative exploration prior to the development of quantitative research plans. Further, qualitative research is often used after quantitative research studies to explore results in more detail and build a rich picture of the findings (Plowright, 2011).

The role of measurement

Measurement is a key tenet of quantitative research, stemming from its logical positivist roots.

In order to assess whether an independent variable has had a significant effect on the dependent variable, both must be objectively measured as accurately as possible. The ultimate goal of quantitative research is the completely objective, valid and reliable measurement of variables and, although in reality this is not often possible, it is the 'gold standard' that should be striven for. This is because it enables the outcome of a study to be generalised to the whole target population and provides external reliability for a study. The level of accuracy desired requires the development of precise tools and techniques to provide high-quality data that can be analysed mathematically or statistically.

Reductionism

In order to explain the assumed reality that is fundamental in quantitative research, researchers often break down complicated systems into smaller parts, or components, that can be measured more easily. These findings may then be used to establish relationships between the parts and provide information about the whole, assuming any generalisation is valid and that the sum of the parts is equal to the whole. It is a way of reducing complex phenomena to universal laws.

Objectivity

Quantitative research is most often based on objective measurements that can be empirically observed, recorded and verified. This is in contrast to qualitative research where the researchers and participants are part of a two-way process that informs understanding as it progresses.

The objectivity in quantitative research is achieved by researchers distinguishing themselves from the subjects they are researching and maintaining a degree of detachment from the research process. This lessens the likelihood that the researchers will influence or bias the outcomes of the research and enhances the probability that the research findings can be replicated by the researchers or other researchers if repeated. The fact that much of the process of developing a quantitative study is transparent – such as the sample design, questionnaire and coding – makes it easier to produce reliable and valid research tools and findings that can be replicated and built on by other researchers. Nevertheless, there are some types of quantitative research where the researchers cannot be as detached from the research as desired – as is the case in observation – and this can introduce researcher bias into these studies.

In a post-positivist framework, quantitative research can be used to collect data relating to human behaviour and emotions that are not easily assessed objectively, such as feelings of depression after counselling. In these cases, the researchers' role is to develop a tool that can collect the information numerically – often a rating scale is developed to meet this need. Such a scale usually consists of categories such as 'much worse', 'neither better nor worse' or 'much better', which effectively reduces subjective assessments to categorical data.

Logico-deductive

Quantitative research is described as 'logico-deductive', meaning that it builds new knowledge on the basis of already existing knowledge using sound arguments. This is in contrast to qualitative research, which is interpretative and builds new knowledge from the findings of each study as it progresses. Using a deductive approach usually involves testing a predetermined idea or hypothesis, to support or reject the proposition.

Data collection

Quantitative research is an umbrella term that covers a wide range of research methods, covered briefly below. Quantitative methods include descriptive, correlational, quasi-experimental and experimental research and, although there are wide variations in these techniques, they are all predetermined, structured and standardised.

Quantitative research tools should be developed prior to the commencement of the data collection process and should not be altered while data are being collected. This ensures that all participants are completing the same tool and data collection is standardised across the group(s). This is equally important whether the tool being developed is a questionnaire, an interview or an observation protocol.

It is also necessary to provide structure to the measurement tool in quantitative research to facilitate the collection of standardised data, such as eye colour, and enable that data to be analysed mathematically. Although open-ended questions *can* be used in gathering quantitative data, they should be used sparingly to ensure that data produced are comparable across the whole sample. Open-ended questions generate varied data, which must be coded if it is to be analysed and this can bring in researcher bias.

While it is important to ensure that the measurement tool is standardised, it is also preferable to try and standardise the setting in which the data is collected, as far as is practical. Thus, administering a questionnaire about how depressed a person feels is likely to achieve very different responses if the person is sitting at home on their own than if he or she is working in a busy office with numerous colleagues to talk to.

Descriptive research

Quantitative research can be used to collect descriptive data from respondents. This can be achieved by means of questionnaires, interviews and observational research. Descriptive research can be used to gain insights into human emotions and opinions by, for example, analysing responses to a questionnaire relating to satisfaction with teaching on a nursing course. It can also be used to understand the frequency of attributes within a population, such as the number of people who prefer red wine or white wine.

Observation is used sometimes in quantitative research although, as is clear from the above, in a different way from how it is used in qualitative research. Whereas in qualitative research it is described and discussed, in quantitative research it usually consists of recording events or actions against a predetermined checklist or rating scale to produce numbers and frequencies of events.

Correlational research

Correlational research aims to systematically investigate and understand the relationships between variables in the real world. It explores linear relationships between two or more variables and determines the types of correlations, positive or negative, and the strength of the relationships. Descriptive studies can often be used to produce data that are analysed in this way.

Experimental and quasi-experimental research

This type of research design is used to measure cause-and-effect relationships between independent and dependent variables and is considered to be the most robust type of quantitative research method. Experimental designs, such as randomised control trials (RCT), have strict 'rules' and employ randomisation and control groups. Quasi-experimental designs may not include randomisation and control and are therefore not as robust, but may be suitable for a wider range of research studies where such strictures are not possible.

Control

It is important in quantitative research to minimise the effects of any extraneous variables – that is, those you are not studying, but which may influence the outcomes – by imposing controls to decrease the risk of error and increase the probability of the results reflecting the reality of a situation as closely as possible.

The level of control varies with the type of study:

- descriptive and correlational research uses minimal controls
- quasi-experimental methods use moderate control
- experimental designs utilise strict controls.

Some of the ways in which control is achieved in quantitative research include the selection of appropriate sampling techniques, randomisation and consistency in the research setting.

Sampling should be used wherever possible to ensure that the selected subjects in the study represent the target population closely. Randomisation helps to reduce bias, minimise the influence of extraneous variables and provide internal validity as all groups are equal at the start of the study. Nevertheless, it is not always cost-effective or viable to use randomisation, so other sampling techniques may need to be employed as appropriate.

CASE STUDY

Gemma wanted to investigate the working practices and roles of students in midwifery departments across the UK. This study was designed as a cross-sectional survey using a postal questionnaire sent to all final year midwifery students in the UK. To ensure that the data could be precisely measured it was vital that the research instrument was valid (measured what it was supposed to measure) and reliable (consistently measured the attributes of interest).

In this study, the questionnaire was designed by a study group of midwifery lecturers and senior midwives. It was piloted with midwifery students who were asked to comment on the clarity of the questionnaire, which was then amended to enhance its face validity.

As it is important that the process of a quantitative study can be replicated, details of the sample population, method of recruitment, use of reminders and response rate were all recorded in the final report. The methods by which the data were collected, entered into a statistical database and analysed, were also provided for transparency and clarity.

The results of the study, based on a 46 per cent response rate, described the role of midwifery students in hospital and highlighted gaps in their knowledge. The survey presented an accurate, nationwide description of the midwifery students and their roles and, due to the robust design and accurate data-gathering methods, the results could be regarded as evidence of the current situation within hospitals.

CONCLUSION

This chapter has given a short overview of quantitative research methodologies. It has described the epistemology, theoretical perspectives and data-collection methods used in quantitative research. Other chapters in the book cover the breadth and variations of on quantitative techniques and some other sources of information are included in the Further Reading and References sections below.

FURTHER READING

Bryman, A. (2012) *Social Research Methods* (4th edn). Oxford: Oxford University Press.
Gerrish, K. and Lacey, A. (eds) (2010) *The Research Process in Nursing* (6th edn). Oxford: Wiley-Blackwell.
Parahoo, K. (2006) *Nursing Research: Principles, process and issues* (2nd edn). Houndmills, Basingstoke and New York: Palgrave Macmillan.

REFERENCES

Bruce, N., Pope, D. and Stanstreet, D. (2008) *Quantitative Methods for Health Research: A practical interactive guide to epidemiology and statistics*. Chichester: John Wiley.
Creswell, J. (2008) *Research Design: Qualitative, quantitative and mixed methods approaches* (3rd edn). Thousand Oaks, CA: Sage.

Creswell, J. and Plano Clark, V. (2007) *Designing and Conducting Mixed Methods Research*. Thousand Oaks, CA: Sage.

Plowright, D. (2011) *Using Mixed Methods: Frameworks for an integrated methodology*. Thousand Oaks, CA: Sage.

Trochim, W. M. (2006) *The Research Methods Knowledge Base* (2nd edn)(available online at: www.socialresearchmethods.net/kb).

7   Mixed Methods Research

Dawn Freshwater and Jane Cahill

DEFINITION

We begin by offering a working definition of mixed methods research (MMR), which will be used as a reference point for this chapter. We would like to highlight that offering a broad definition of MMR is a challenge, given the diversity of philosophical and epistemological assumptions that researchers bring to their definitions and understandings of this concept. For the purposes of this chapter, however, we shall define MMR as a research design with philosophical assumptions and quantitative and qualitative methods (Creswell and Plano Clark, 2011). The advantages to researchers of this approach are numerous and wide-ranging, the main ones being that mixing methods enhances the validity of a study (by providing multiple methods, perspectives and data sets to examine the phenomenon in question), results in richer data and fosters creative and innovative ways of conducting methodological inquiries.

KEY POINTS

- Definitions of MMR are determined by whether mixed methods writers consider this form of research as a methodology or a method
- As a methodology, the MMR design builds on philosophical assumptions that researchers use to guide them in the collection, analysis and synthesis of data throughout the research process
- As a method, the MMR design also provides guidance on how to collect, analyse and synthesise quantitative and qualitative data in a single study or series of studies

- MMR provides a fuller understanding of a research question or phenomenon than either the qualitative or the quantitative approach alone. The use of both approaches is believed to enhance the external validity of the MMR design (Bryman, 2004)
- Between methods triangulation in MMR can also mitigate against bias (observer, measurement) possible when one approach alone is used. MMR has the potential to mitigate the effects of the sometimes conflicting relationship between qualitative and quantitative researchers
- The MMR design contains both qualitative and quantitative components and typically the design evolves in the process of the research being undertaken (Tashakkori and Creswell, 2007)
- Synthesising or 'mixing' is central to the definition of MMR. Data need to be mixed in a way that will provide a fuller understanding of the research question or the phenomenon under investigation than if a single approach (quantitative or qualitative) had been used
- Morse defines a mixed method design in Johnson et al. (2007) as a plan for a scientifically rigorous research process comprised of qualitative (QUAL) or quantitative (QUAN) *core component* that directs the theoretical drive, with qualitative (QUAL) or quantitative (QUAN) *supplementary component(s)* (QUAL/QUAN + QUAL/QUAN)
- There is a debate in the mixed methods community as to whether MMR constitutes a paradigm in its own right or it is simply a choice of methods within paradigm(s) (Creswell, 2011; Denzin, 2010)

DISCUSSION

Definitions

Definitions of MMR are determined by whether researchers view this approach as a 'method' or a 'methodology'. We define 'methodology' as a philosophical framework that guides the methods used throughout the process of research and 'method' as the techniques of data collection, analysis and synthesis.

There are differences among those in the MMR community as to how MMR is understood and this continues to be an important debate. Those who view MMR as a *methodology* focus on the philosophical assumptions they bring to their mode of enquiry in all phases of the research process (Freshwater, 2007; Mertens, 2007; Tashakkori and Teddlie, 2003, 2010). While some argue that this introduces a complexity, it is important to be mindful that researchers should be aware of the implicit assumptions or worldviews that influence how they conduct their research. Those who view MMR as a *method* focus on the methods employed to collect, analyse and interpret combinations of qualitative and quantitative data. (Creswell et al., 2003; Onwuegbuzie and Teddlie, 2003). Understanding MMR as a method appeals to some researchers because it is clean and concise (Elliot, 2005).

Design issues

Synthesising or 'mixing' is central to the principles of MMR. Mixing the data sets provides a fuller understanding of the research question than the use of either of these data sets alone. Mixing can occur in three ways:

- the merging or converging of the data sets
- connecting the two data sets, so one set builds on the other, serving an additive function
- nesting one data set within the other, so one a set provides a supportive role for the other.

Advantages of MMR

It is generally acknowledged that the value of MMR lies in its ability to provide more complete evidence on a research question than would be provided by one approach alone. This argument is commonly put forward to promote the external validity of the MMR design.

One design that is very well known in MMR and supports external validity issues is the 'triangulation design' (Bryman, 2004; Creswell et al., 2003), the purpose of which is to gather 'different and complementary data on the same topic' (Morse, 1991: 122). The triangulation design helps to enhance the reliability of the MMR approach by mitigating bias introduced by the use of one approach alone. Denzin (1978: 14) claims that 'the bias inherent in any particular data source, investigators, and particularly method will be cancelled out when used in conjunction with other data sources, investigators, and methods'.

MMR designs bring together the strong and weak characteristics of quantitative designs (large sample sizes, trends, the ability to generalise from results, weak in understanding the context setting) and qualitative designs (small numbers, in depth, researcher bias), thereby offsetting the bias introduced by one approach alone and building on the collective strengths of the approaches.

The paradigm debate

There is some debate within the MMR community as to whether or not MMR constitutes a conceptually distinct paradigm (or worldview).

One school of thought, exemplified by Mertens (2007, 2010) conceptualises paradigms as sets of philosophical assumptions relating to the nature of methodology, epistemology, ontology and axiology. According to this model, methodological assumptions can lead to a choice of mixed methods within several paradigms, most notably the pragmatic and transformative paradigms, although mixed methods does not constitute a paradigm itself.

There is another school of thought that allows for paradigms to be methodological in their foundation. This line of thinking is exemplified by writers such as Denscombe (2008) and Johnson and Onwuegbuzie (2004), who have conceptualised the mixed methods approach as a third paradigm for social research in the way they combine quantitative and qualitative methodologies (see also Freshwater and Cahill, 2012).

CASE STUDY

For this section, in which we demonstrate how the principles of MMR can be applied in healthcare, we cite an ongoing, externally funded research project that is being led in the UK by the first author of this chapter. It is a pioneering theory and evidence-based programme and represents a collaborative venture between the School of Healthcare at the University of Leeds, NSPCC, the Anna Freud Centre and leading researchers at Yale University.

The aims of this study are to evaluate an intensive programme of home visiting of disadvantaged, young, first-time mothers and their infants. Healthcare professionals will support its effectiveness by promoting secure attachment, parental reflectiveness and self-efficacy.

The team in Yale has been delivering the programme for several years and has been tracking babies who have been involved with this programme for the first five years of their lives. The team's evaluation of this longitudinal study employs mixed methods. The Minding the Baby (MTB) programme evaluation is an efficacy study – that is, a randomised controlled trial in which mother and infant dyads are assigned to the intervention group (MTB programme alongside standard care) or control group (standard prenatal, postpartum and paediatric primary care and monthly educational materials about child health and development). The evaluation includes quantitative analyses of maternal and infant outcome variables (including a cost-effectiveness analysis) and detailed qualitative analyses of transcribed pregnancy and parent development interviews that describe the evolution of the respective reflective capacities of adolescent mothers in the intervention and control groups.

CONCLUSION

The business of research, like any other business, has to move with and adapt to the changing environment. The first author's experience as an editor of an international impact-factored journal located within the health disciplines for over 9 years, along with both authors' research careers spanning 20 years, have provided us with wide-ranging methodological insights and the ability to see the potential impact of research outcomes on population health, clinical practice, academic education and research protocols. For this reason, it is timely to consider the specific impacts of MMR in nursing and healthcare.

The global economic and environmental climate at the time of writing raises concerns for the future funding of research and highlights the absolute need to demonstrate the impact and outcomes of our research studies and, indeed, our theoretical and philosophical deliberations that go on to inform research design. There is emerging evidence that available funding is more readily accessible for those who are willing and able to facilitate successful interdisciplinary collaborations and also willing to recognise the relative merits and limitations of a variety of approaches to achieve the same ends and appreciate the coexistence of multiple truths. For example, Plano Clark (2010), in a study of US trends in federally funded health-related research, observes that mixed methods projects are being funded and makes recommendations for impacting the dynamic relationship between researchers' decisions to use mixed methods and existing funding mechanisms. In the UK, the Medical Research Council's methodology research programme includes in its remit the development of 'methodologies in the applied disciplines underpinning research in the health sciences, for example ... qualitative analysis and mixed methods' (Medical Research Council, 2013).

Viewing a phenomenon or research question through multiple lenses is, we believe, a good image for MMR, an image that encourages researchers to embrace the methodological rigour of synthesising diverse sources of evidence and cultivate an awareness of how evidence will, in a sense, always be a partial truth contingent on the methodological line of enquiry employed by the researcher. We hope this chapter, with its inclusion of a working definition, highlighting key points and an inspirational example of a mixed methods research project that has an impact, has provided a good starting point for researchers wishing to enter the still emergent field of mixed methods research.

FURTHER READING

Creswell, J.W. and Plano Clark, V.L. (2011) *Designing and Conducting Mixed Methods Research* (2nd edn). Thousand Oaks, CA: Sage.

Tashakkori, A. and Teddlie, C. (eds) (2010) *SAGE Handbook of Mixed Methods in Social and Behavioural Research* (2nd edn). Thousand Oaks, CA: Sage.

REFERENCES

Bryman, A. (2004) 'Methods Briefing 11: Integrating quantitative and qualitative research'. University of Leicester: Leicester.

Creswell, J.W. (2011) 'Controversies in mixed methods research', in J.W. Creswell and V.L. Plano Clark, *Designing and Conducting Mixed Methods Research* (2nd edn). Thousand Oaks, CA: Sage. pp. 269–83.

Creswell, J.W., Plano Clark, V.L., Gutmann, M.L. and Hanson, W.E. (2003) 'Advanced mixed methods research designs', in A. Tashakkori and C. Teddlie (eds), *Handbook of Mixed Methods in Social and Behavioural Research*. Thousand Oaks, CA: Sage. pp. 209–40.

Denscombe, M. (2008) 'Communities of practice: A research paradigm for the mixed methods approach', *Journal of Mixed Methods Research*, 2: 270–83.

Denzin, N.K. (2010) 'Moments, mixing methods and paradigm dialogs', *Qualitative Inquiry*, 16 (6): 419–27.

Denzin, N.K. (1978) *The Research Act: A theoretical introduction to sociological methods*. New York: McGraw-Hill.

Elliot, J. (2005) *Using Narrative in Social Research: Qualitative and quantitative approaches*. London: Sage.

Freshwater, D. (2007) 'Reading mixed methods research: Contexts for criticism', *Journal of Mixed Methods Research*, 1 (2): 134–46.

Freshwater, D. and Cahill, J. (2012) 'Why write?', *Journal of Mixed Methods Research*, 6 (3): 151–3.

Johnson, R.B. and Onwuegbuzie, A.J. (2004) 'Mixed methods research: A research paradigm whose time has come', *Educational Researcher*, 33: 14–26.

Johnson, R.B., Onwuegbuzie, A.J. and Turner, L.A. (2007) 'Toward a definition of mixed methods research', *Journal of Mixed Methods Research*, 1 (2): 112–33.

Medical Research Council (2013) Methodology research programme. Available at: http://www.mrc.ac.uk/Ourresearch/ResearchInitiatives/MRP/index.htm (accessed 28 May 2013).

Mertens, D.M. (2007) 'Transformative paradigm: Mixed methods and social justice', *Journal of Mixed Methods Research*, 1: 212–25.

Mertens, D.M. (2010). 'Transformative mixed methods research', *Qualitative Inquiry*, 16: 469–74.

Morse, J.M. (1991) 'Approaches to qualitative–quantitative methodological triangulation', *Nursing Research*, 40: 120–23.

Onwuegbuzie, A.J. and Teddlie, C. (2003) 'A framework for analyzing data in mixed methods research', in A. Tashakkori and C. Teddlie (eds), *Handbook of Mixed Methods in Social and Behavioural Research*. Thousand Oaks, CA: Sage. pp. 351–83.

Plano Clark, V.L. (2010) 'The adoption and practice of mixed methods: U.S. trends in federally funded health-related research', *Qualitative Inquiry*, 16: 428–40.

Tashakkori, A. and Creswell, J. (2007) 'Exploring the nature of research questions in mixed methods research', *Journal of Mixed Methods Research*, 1 (3): 207–11.

Tashakkori, A. and Teddlie, C. (eds) (2003) *Handbook of Mixed Methods in Social and Behavioural Research*. Thousand Oaks, CA: Sage.

Tashakkori, A. and Teddlie, C. (eds) (2010) *Sage Handbook of Mixed Methods in Social and Behavioral Research* (2nd edn). Thousand Oaks, CA: Sage.

8 Evaluation Research

David Coyle

DEFINITION

Within the context of research, some may find evaluation being allocated to a separate category of study surprising. Surely any form of enquiry is making a decision about an event, situation or action? What makes evaluation within this context different is that where some methods seek to manipulate and control factors for testing hypotheses and other approaches explore the moment for an individual or group, evaluative research is interested in what happens in the real world when something new is tried. As Bryman (2008: 693) succinctly states that the definition of evaluation research is 'research that is concerned with the evaluation of real-life interventions in the social world'.

KEY POINTS

- Evaluation research is used by many different stakeholders across the public and private sectors
- It is set in the real world and focuses on change occurring therein

- The method supports experimental, quasi-experimental, survey, consumer satisfaction, clinical audit, educational standards and other regulatory functions
- Quality in evaluation research depends on turning a value statement into a factual standard

DISCUSSION

Deciding on when a study should involve evaluation methods usually centres on whether or not undertaking a different or more positivist approach would raise too many ethical or practical obstacles. Evaluative research fills that gap, providing policymakers and theory generators with a powerful approach that is flexible and potentially robust.

By placing the approach within the real world, evaluation research automatically has a positivist view. The belief that the world can be understood and studied externally is a part of the evaluation method. Within realism, however, two broad schools exist:

- one aims to understand reality provided appropriate tools are used
- in the other reality may be mediated via the observations of the researcher or just be an observation (Bryman, 2008).

Evaluation research is everywhere and used by many different stakeholders. It may be called by various names and employ a vast range of methodological techniques. Such breadth is one of the method's strengths, in that the tenets may be applied across diverse settings. Of course, with such flexibility comes the potential for weakness. Anyone could engage in evaluation or ask a series of questions, but, as Clarke (1999: 2) clearly states:

> Evaluation is presented as a form of applied social research, the primary purpose of which is not to discover new knowledge, as is the case with basic research, but to study the effectiveness with which existing knowledge is used to inform practical action.

The key to understanding whether evaluation research is good or not lies in whether or not the evaluation criteria are good. A simple question – 'What is good?' – but the answer depends on who is asking it and what the aim of the proposed evaluation is. Evaluation must have at its heart the question of whether or not the intervention/innovation or status quo is effective. In other words, is whatever we are doing working? This view is echoed by many (Brophy et al., 2008; Clark, 1999; Patton, 2001).

In order to overcome what is called 'value bias', criteria for the evaluation should be set. If the proposed evaluation is a government department interested in getting a better idea of whether or not a new policy or change is profitable within its manifesto, then questions about cost, effectiveness and profitability may be more important than other implications of the proposed change. Were the evaluation commissioned instead by a charity that worked with homeless people who may well be affected by the government's proposal, one can see the questions would be different. As Brophy et al. (2008) remind us, an evaluation project cannot ask and answer every question each stakeholder may have in any given project.

Gomm (2009) makes the point that sometimes researchers will be provided with evaluation criteria as part of the contract and they are to act as a specification. The commissioning party may undertake some work in developing a set of evaluation criteria. Gomm (2009) also states that often an agency or service will seek an evaluation and evaluation criteria from a person with knowledge and expertise within the area under consideration; this is the case in the study presented below.

Bryman (2008: 381) cites Spencer et al.'s (2003) work for the government of the day determining the quality of evaluation research. Bryman cites its use for deciding on structurally robust evaluation research within a qualitative framework, but also highlights the dichotomy of confining qualitative methodology to a checklist, even if it forms part of a larger framework.

Table 8.1 shows a sound framework where a theme of good enquiry is shown and any evaluative study adhering to it would be of use.

Clarke (1999: 5) makes a good distinction between *evaluation* and *audit*, in which he cites Clemisky (1985), that audit and evaluation may share some similarities, with the former focusing on 'normative questions' rather than descriptive or cause and effect ones.

Table 8.1   Framework for evaluation research

1. How credible are the findings?	2. Has knowledge/understanding be extended by the research?
3. How well does the evaluation address its original aims and purposes?	4. Scope for drawing wider influences – how well is this explained?
5. How clear is the basis for the evaluation appraisal?	6. How defensible is the research design?
7. How well defended is the sample design/ target selection or cases/documents?	8. Sample composition/case inclusion – how well is the eventual composition described?
9. How well has the data collection been carried out?	10. How well has the approach to, and formulation of, the analysis been conveyed?
11. Context of data sources – how well are they retained and portrayed?	12. How well have diversity of perspective and content been explored?
13. How well has detail, depth and complexity (richness) of the data been conveyed?	14. How clear are the links between data, interpretation and conclusion – that is, how well can the route to any conclusions be seen?
15. How clear and coherent is the reporting?	16. How clear are the assumptions/theoretical perspectives/values that have shaped the form and output of the evaluation?
17. What evidence is there of attention to ethical issues?	18. How adequately has the research process been documented?

One feature of evaluation research Gomm (2009: 332) bravely highlights is that, anecdotally, many evaluative researchers' final reports present a 'sympathetic bias' towards the innovation, 'omitting criticisms from their written reports' and, instead, confidentially providing a less positive view to the commissioners. Gomm points out that, therefore, those reading reports of evaluation research should do so carefully, especially if they are planning to replicate the innovation or project.

CASE STUDY

A small-scale project established a small-scale personalisation pilot in a metropolitan authority substance misuse service over a 12-month period. It explored the impact and outcomes of people misusing substances receiving an individual budget for part of their treatment. Individual budgets are mandatory in social care settings and are being promoted in healthcare. For groups of people whose addictions and behaviour place them both at the periphery of society and in contact with the criminal justice system, however, any change in service approach should be seen within an evaluation research frame.

The research group was commissioned to assist in the design of the service innovation process and identify suitable approaches to assist in the development of the pilot. The project sought to explore three themes.

Objectives

1. To explore the experience, a small cohort of service users, at different points along the timeline of their treatment, were offered an individual budget.

   This arm of the evaluation aimed to recruit a cohort of individuals accessing addiction services in a metropolitan authority who had agreed to take part in the virtual individual budget pilot. A case study design was employed and service users were selected to represent two different treatment durations. Equal numbers of individual budget recipients were sought at commencement of their contact with the service at approximately 36 or more months. The timings were important and set by the commissioning group as 36 or more months of methadone use had a poorer prognosis for change than earlier withdrawal. Each person completed a survey tool in addition to two interviews over the duration of the innovation. A narrative frame was used in analysis and in addition to textural analysis software. Each person recruited was subject to a full consent process on the basis that participation was entirely voluntary and without prejudice.

2. To explore and analyse the service providers' experience and perception of individual budgets.

   Focus groups were scheduled at two points for service workers from a range of agencies, such as health, probation and community safety. The nature of the agencies' work and limitations of time, however, meant the investigators utilised a reflexive approach and instead focused on interviews (face to face or by telephone) with key informants approximately two thirds through the evaluation. Each interview was transcribed and subject to textural analysis software.

3. To calculate the relative costs of individual budgets for services using data from current costings.

    The final element to this evaluation involved a simple cost comparison of documentary data sources available from the commissioner.

The design aimed to capture a developing picture of change for service users at different stages of their contact with health services, encompassing a range of stakeholders. The study was reflexive and, while mostly qualitative, sought to also utilise survey and comparative statistics. A critical realist perspective shows that, while the evaluators had sympathy with the innovation on the basis of their previous work, they were sensitive to culture and the difficulties of implementing the innovation in this contentious setting. The challenge with a project of this nature was to attempt to listen with parity to *all* stakeholders and maintain a direction for the study in an ever-changing landscape.

CONCLUSION

Whether the evaluation is research for the research community or for service providers identifying the effectiveness of their work or part of an audit, for example, the process of asking what is the worth of something is paramount. In healthcare, every service will have as part of its mission that the hospital, clinic or agency will seek to provide a safe, effective and caring system for the benefit of all its users.

    That would be true if, in fact, it happened. The above statement is an aspiration, a value or a hope. As the report of the Mid Stafford NHS Foundation Trust's public inquiry, chaired by Robert Francis (Stationery Office, 2013), with its 290 recommendations for improving the National Health Service in England painfully pointed out, rhetoric does not always equal reality. Therefore, it is essential that, when formulating evaluation research, care is given to the process of determining what is under scrutiny and how the researchers will recognise what is being evaluated. It is essential that, where evaluation is undertaken, it is done to determine the merit of what is being attempted by those qualified to make a judgement and the design of the study/process elicits robust information understood by those responsible and, as stated in all evaluation research, acted on to change the status quo.

FURTHER READING

Brophy, S., Snooks, H. and Griffiths, L. (2008) *Small-scale Evaluation in Health: A practical handbook*. London: Sage.
Patton, M.Q. (2001) *Qualitative Research and Evaluation Methods* (3rd edn) London: Sage.

REFERENCES

Brophy, S., Snooks, H. and Griffiths, L. (2008) *Small-scale Evaluation in Health: A practical handbook*. London: Sage.
Bryman, A. (2008) *Social Research Methods* (3rd edn). Oxford: Oxford University Press.

Clarke, F. (1999) *Evaluation Research: An introduction to principles, methods and practice.* London: Sage.

Gomm, R. (2009) *Social Research Methodology* (2nd edn). Houndmills, Basingstoke: Palgrave Macmillan.

Francis, R. (2013) 'Mid Stafford NHS Foundation Trust Public Inquiry'. London: The Stationery Office.

Patton, M.Q. (2001) *Qualitative Research and Evaluation Methods* (3rd edn). London: Sage.

9 Service User-Led Research

Aidan Worsley

DEFINITION

There are various definitional issues attached to the concept of 'service user-led research' – not least the notion that 'service user' is itself a contested concept – but it is where we must begin because it is fundamental to the constructions of research possibly attaching to such a group.

When we think of the term 'service users', we might think of carers, patients, people who used to receive services, and it will be used in this chapter to include all these groups. Broadly speaking, it will be used to mean people who are users of services provided along the health and social care spectrum.

Of course, the term 'service user' also inherently limits our conception of any particular person as it reduces them to a relationship with a service – failing to capture the fact that such a relationship may be relatively inconsequential in their lives. Talking of mere 'entitlement' to services can also mask the unequal relationships that many service users experience in society – unemployment, poor housing, problems of access and so on. This disadvantage appears to be replicated to some extent in research in the health and social care arena. While such research has come to involve more and more users of services, it has often been in tokenistic and/or relatively minor roles. Research largely remains something 'done *to*' service users rather than something 'done *by*' them, but this is changing, as Evans and Jones (2004: 8) note:

> So, what is entailed in user-led research? Essentially it is about service users determining the research focus, the research process, the interpretation of the findings, and the conclusions to be drawn for practice and policy.

It is this fundamental shift in orientation that will be explored here and some critical illustrations of service user-led research will also be provided.

KEY POINTS

- The involvement of service users in research exists along a spectrum of consultation, collaboration and control
- There are relatively few examples of service user-led research in health and social care
- This kind of research often focuses on the lives and experiences of users themselves and seeks social change

DISCUSSION

One of the interesting questions with which to begin this discussion is, 'Who gets researched?' A simple answer may be 'The less powerful'. As Oliver (1992: 110) notes, 'research tends to focus on the poor, the unemployed, the sick and disabled'. It has uncovered relatively little about psychiatrists, politicians, policymakers and, even, researchers themselves. Indeed, there is relatively little research on nurses and social workers, for example, when compared to the volume investigating the disadvantaged groups noted above.

The social distance that exists between service users and researchers is significant. Research is associated with – and primarily takes place within – an academic or clinical environment. There is a significant body of evidence for the notion that service users struggle to 'fit in' to academic structures and settings (see, for example, Branfield, 2007). This struggle to bridge the gap is a recurring theme in social research, with challenges in methodological, process and political arenas.

There are some methodological approaches that provide a pathway towards service user-led research.

- 'Participatory action research' (PAR) considers people's lived experiences as a starting point for research, tending to emphasise social change, authentic participation and collaboration.
- 'Feminist research methodology' (a very broad umbrella) tends to be critical of traditional ('malestream') research practices, often done by men, focusing on men and producing a masculine version of the word that is applied to the whole population. Research, it is typically argued from this perspective, needs to focus more on the individual, 'the personal is political' and, thus, of course, the relationship between researcher and researched becomes a central issue, as do the daily lives of people, their thoughts and feelings.
- 'Emancipatory research', the disabled people's research movement, and 'survivor research' (linked to psychiatric systems) approaches form a struggle against the traditional medicalisation and clinical bias of research. Individualised research in these approaches reinforces a model of, for example,

disability that presumes the problems of disability are caused by individual impairments rather than more social issues. Thus, the problems one has at work as a disabled person are reframed as the problems work gives one through inadequacies in the physical environment and the attitudes of others (Oliver, 1992). Survivor research is used to capture both the experiences of those surviving the experience of mental health problems and their treatment and engagement with mental health services. Survivor research argues that the subjective nature of mental health problems means that it is survivors who should lead and define research about themselves – to provide greater insight into their needs and more accurately identify their views and experiences of services, support and treatment. Furthermore, the control of research agendas is an empowering component for survivors (Hardwick and Worsley, 2011).

Where these approaches and the very notion of service user-led research challenge traditional research most is perhaps in their embracing of the moral, ethical and subjective elements of social research. This, of course, clashes with positivist constructions of research and its quest for objectivity. Service user-led research strives for social change, not simply for objective knowledge. It seeks to improve people's lives; its emphasis is on empowerment. If we posit Becker's (1967) question, 'Whose side are we on?', service user-led research is very much on the side of the service user.

Some of the examples that do exist point to a way forward. Middleton et al.'s (2011) research involved service users being trained as researchers and conducting the research themselves – in this case, into the effectiveness of crisis resolution home treatment, but also exploring the limitations of positivist approaches in exploring mental health difficulties.

Tischler et al. (2010) involved patients in examining the extent and results of patient-centeredness in a wide range of existing schizophrenia research projects. They showed that patient-centred research had many benefits in terms of the quality of the research and was highly valued by patients and doctors alike.

Wilson et al. (2010) describe the development of a mental health service user- and carer-led research group in a university setting, providing training and developing user-led research projects.

CASE STUDY

When we start to operationalise the notion of service user-led research – and ask ourselves how we (as academic or practitioner researchers) might facilitate this – a range of challenges swiftly emerge. Not least of these is the problem of 'letting go'.

If the research is led by service users, then the academic researcher is, by definition, in a different role from that usually expected – perhaps one of supporter and facilitator. Particularly as academic researchers are skilled in research methodology, the notion of giving such 'expert power' away in this kind of process is challenging.

The aims, objectives, design, conduct, analysis and dissemination of the research should be determined and controlled by the service users. We might, though, see debates concerning the suitability of service users to taking on these tasks across a number of contexts. At what age can children and young people take on a research role? How can we involve people with learning disabilities in the research process? Perhaps there are some kinds of service users who ought to be excluded from involvement – certain types of offenders, for example? Are there certain types of illness, disability, language barriers and so on that mean some people can't lead research?

The case study in this brief chapter gives an illustration from just one of these groups. It looks at how a group of people with learning disabilities led a piece of research – a group who shared a view with those we have outlined above regarding traditional forms of research and, indeed, support (Taylor et al., 2008: 28):

> Jennifer has explained why we are doing this research. … People like psychiatrists and doctors and teachers and stuff are writing stuff about us saying that we are stupid and can't do stuff, but we are not stupid. We've got our own minds. We know what's good for us and we know what we want in our lives, not them telling us what we want in our lives. They're the ones who are wrong.

The project was led by People First Lambeth, with support from the Shaping Our Lives Network, Brunel University and Trust for London.

Beginning from perspective of service users, with service users as researchers, the group wanted to write about the things that they cared about most and what was happening in their lives, which included (Taylor et al., 2008: 19):

- people going to day centres and not getting properly paid jobs
- people being nasty to people with learning difficulties and making them feel stupid
- people with learning difficulties being controlled or bossed around by people without learning difficulties.

The report examines these and other issues in a direct and candid manner, having a significant emotional impact on readers as the research allows a connection with the authors' experiences, stories and lives. One participant sums up what was something of a general view of people with learning difficulties (Taylor et al., 2008: 90):

> I don't like it when organisations say they are going to involve people with learning difficulties and they don't involve us in things about us. I don't like it when people get big money and don't give people with learning difficulties any of the money to work with them. I don't like the way people don't ask us. They say they ask us here but they done it before. I don't like when they get funding bids, and this is big money, big money, and they don't ask us if we want to be part of the training.

CONCLUSION

Service user-led research in health and social care is still, in the main, a disappointingly rare occurrence. Indeed, McLaughlin (2007) calls it the 'next frontier'. More often, we see varying levels of service user involvement in research projects. Arnstein's (1971) early work in this area is a useful tool for assessing the gradients between consultation, collaboration and control.

Of course, different research projects call for different approaches, but researchers are encouraged to reflect carefully on the benefits of service user involvement and, indeed, ask themselves whether or not they are able to act as support to service user-led research when engaged in the generation of knowledge that affect lives other than their own.

FURTHER READING

Taylor, J., Williams, V., Johnson, R., Hiscut, I. and Brennan, M. (2008) *We Are Not Stupid*. London: People First Lambeth and Shaping Our Lives (available online at: www.shapingourlives.org.uk/downloads/publications/wearenotstupid.pdf).

Wilson, C., Fothergill, A. and Rees, H. (2010) 'A potential model for the first all Wales mental health service user- and care-led research group', *Journal of Psychiatric and Mental Health Nursing*, 17: 31–8.

REFERENCES

Arnstein, S. (1971) 'A ladder of citizen participation', *Journal of the Royal Planning Institute*, 35 (4): 216–24.

Becker, H. (1967) 'Whose side are we on?', *Social Problems*, 14 (Winter): 239–47.

Branfield, F. (2007) 'User involvement in social work education: Report of regional consultations with service users to develop a strategy to support the participation of service users in social work education'. Swindon: Shaping Our Lives National User Network.

Evans, C. and Jones, R. (2004) 'Engagement and empowerment, research and relevance: Comments on user-controlled research', *Research, Policy and Planning*, 22 (2): 5–13.

Hardwick, L. and Worsley, A. (2011) *Doing Social Work Research*. London: Sage.

McLaughlin, H. (2007) *Understanding Social Work Research*. London: Sage.

Middleton, H., Shaw, R., Collier, R., Purser, A. and Ferguson, B. (2011) 'The dodo bird verdict and the elephant in the room: A service user-led investigation of crisis resolution and home treatment', *Health Sociology Review*, 20 (2): 147–56.

Oliver, M. (1992) 'Changing the social relations of research production?', *Disability and Society*, 7 (2): 101–14.

Taylor, J., Williams, V., Johnson, R., Hiscut, I. and Brennan, M. (2008) *We Are Not Stupid*. London: People First Lambeth and Shaping Our Lives (available online at: www.shapingourlives.org.uk/downloads/publications/wearenotstupid.pdf).

Tischler, V., D'Silva, K., Cheetham, A., Goring, M. and Calton, T. (2010) 'Involving patients in research: The challenge of patient-centeredness', *International Journal of Social Psychiatry*, 56 (6): 623–63.

Wilson, C., Fothergill, A. and Rees, H. (2010) 'A potential model for the first all Wales mental health service user- and care-led research group', *Journal of Psychiatric and Mental Health Nursing*, 17: 31–8.

10 Systematic Reviews

Alan Pearson

DEFINITION

A 'systematic review' aims to provide a comprehensive and unbiased summary of the best available evidence on a single topic, bringing together multiple individual studies in a single document. As part of the systematic review process, individual research studies are subjected to critical appraisal. Systematic reviews thus provide evidence for clinical decision-making, as well as identifying future research needs.

The risk of human error during the review process is minimised by having two or more people undertake the critical appraisal and data extraction. As a result of these processes, however, systematic reviews are time-consuming and expensive.

The process of conducting a systematic review is a scientific exercise and, as the results influence healthcare decisions, it is important to apply the same degree of rigour as that expected in primary research. The quality of a review, and its recommendations, depends on the extent to which scientific review methods are followed to minimise the risk of error and bias. These explicit and rigorous methods differentiate systematic reviews from traditional reviews of literature (JBI, 2011).

KEY POINTS

The key characteristics of a systematic review are (Green et al., 2008: 6):

- a clearly stated set of objectives with predefined eligibility criteria for the studies
- an explicit, reproducible methodology
- a systematic search that attempts to identify all studies meeting the eligibility criteria
- an assessment of the validity of the findings of the included studies – for example, via the assessment of the risk of bias
- a systematic presentation, and synthesis, of the characteristics and findings of the included studies

DISCUSSION

A systematic review is a form of research; indeed, it is frequently referred to as 'secondary research' as it reviews primary research ('primary research' involves designing and conducting a study). A systematic review also collects and analyses data, but usually from published and unpublished reports of completed research.

The first step in a systematic review is the development of a 'proposal' or 'protocol'. Protocol development begins with a search of databases, such as the Cochrane Database of Systematic Reviews. If the topic of the protocol has not been the subject of a systematic review, then a new review protocol is developed and submitted for peer review and publication.

The review question

The protocol should state the questions that will be pursued in the review. Questions should be specific regarding the population, setting, interventions or phenomena and outcomes of interest.

The review protocol

Systematic reviewers develop a protocol and subject it to peer review before commencing the review itself. Once a protocol is finalised, it is lodged in an online database so that other reviewers interested in a given topic can search these databases to avoid duplication of reviews.

The review protocol provides a predetermined plan to ensure scientific rigour. It also allows for periodic updating of the review if necessary. Updating systematic reviews is imperative in a climate of continuous information production. As new research knowledge is generated on a regular basis, updates of systematic reviews are essential in order to ensure that health practices are based on current research evidence. Updates are usually carried out on a three- to five-year cycle, depending on the topic.

A number of decisions critical to the quality of the systematic review are made. For example, when a systematic review seeks to utilise multiple forms of research, the review criteria will be different from those associated with a review of research involving only quantitative data. There are standard criteria, however, that are addressed in the protocol. Every effort should be made to adhere to the criteria set in the protocol, although, as with primary research, there may be instances where changes are unavoidable. Any such changes should be declared in the final review report.

CASE STUDY

Hussain chose to submit a systematic review for his dissertation. He used the template shown in Table 10.1 as a guide for his review protocol.

Hussain referred to the following notes to guide his review.

Background review

The background for a systematic review includes:

- a discussion of the review question and how it emerged
- an assessment of the significance of the topic to healthcare
- an overview of the issues relevant to the review question
- an overview of previous reviews of the review topic or of topics related to it
- a description of any controversies related to the review topic.

Table 10.1 Systematic review protocol template

Example of a systematic review protocol	
Title:	The title of a review will be drawn from the question that reviewers are seeking to answer
Background:	
Objectives:	
Criteria for considering studies for this review:	Types of participants
	Types of intervention
	Types of outcome measures
	Types of studies
Search strategy for identification of studies:	
Methods of the review:	Selecting studies for inclusion
	Assessment of quality
	Methods used to collect data from included studies
	Methods used to synthesise data
	Date review to commence
	Date review to be completed

It is equally important to justify why elements are *not* included. In describing the background literature, value statements about the effect of interventions should be avoided. Existing research results may be conflicting, variations in current practice may be identified or potential gaps in the body of research may be motivating factors. The background provides a clear and logical progression to your review question.

Objectives

Objectives for the review can best be illustrated by example. In a review entitled 'The effectiveness of mechanical compression devices in attaining hemostasis after removal of a femoral sheath following femoral artery cannulation for cardiac interventional procedures: A systematic review' (Jones, 2000), the objective was stated in the following way:

The main objective of this review was to present the best available information on the effectiveness of mechanical compression devices in achieving hemostasis after removal of the femoral sheath from patients after cardiac interventions.

Inclusion criteria

The protocol describes the criteria used to select the literature. These might be:

- the types of studies to be included (for example, randomised controlled trials, pseudo-randomised controlled trials or interpretative studies)
- the intervention, activity or phenomenon (for example, pharmaceutical and non-pharmaceutical interventions for smoking cessation)

- the outcome (for example, smoking cessation or reduction)
- the specific study populations (for example, adult males aged 18 years and over who have been smoking for at least 5 years)
- language of publication (for example, English only or English, German, Spanish and Japanese)
- the time period (for example, study reports published or made available between 2007 and 2013).

Search strategy

It is important to develop a thorough search strategy, if poorly structured, it can diminish the quality of the review, should it not identify research papers pertinent to your review question. The protocol provides a detailed strategy that will be used to identify all relevant literature within an agreed timeframe. To identify all relevant studies for the review, the search strategy included searches of:

- indexes of periodical articles (such as CINAHL, MEDLINE/PubMed)
- indexes of reports, theses and conference papers (such as Dissertation Abstracts and Conference Papers Index)
- Major sources of evidence-based practice information (such as the Cochrane Collaboration)
- websites of nursing and midwifery organisations and other relevant agencies (such as MIRIAD).

It is important to contact experts in the field to ensure the relevant studies are included. In this case, relevant studies with an English language abstract were located for assessment against the inclusion criteria.

Assessment criteria

The protocol describes how the validity of primary studies will be assessed and any exclusion criteria based on quality considerations.

Data extraction

It is necessary to extract data from the primary research regarding the participants, intervention, outcome measures and results. Accurate and consistent data extraction is important and often data extraction forms are utilised to achieve this. Examples of sheets developed for this purpose should be included as part of the protocol.

Data synthesis

It is important to combine the literature in an appropriate manner when producing a report. Statistical analysis (meta-analysis) or textual analysis (meta-synthesis) may or may not be used and will depend on the nature and quality of studies included in the review. While it may not be possible to state exactly what analysis will be undertaken, the general approach should be included in the protocol.

Hussain has submitted his systematic review and now, with his supervisor's guidance, is preparing a paper for publication based on his work.

CONCLUSION

Whenever health professionals engage in practice, they make clinical decisions and draw on a wide range of evidence. This will include knowledge of the basic biological and behavioural sciences, the health professionals' assessments of the current context and individual patients, as well as their own experience and current understandings of research reports that they may have read. All of the knowledge that is used to make clinical decisions can be referred to as evidence – and the validity of this evidence may be variable.

The assumption of a systematic review is that there are things we need to know in order to conduct our practice professionally, but there are substantial gaps in the knowledge available to us. It aims to expose the gaps in specific areas and provide pointers to the kinds of questions to which we need to find answers.

Although health professionals often want to answer broad questions, the narrower a question is, the easier it is to conduct the review and the more useful the final product will be. If the reviewers are interested in finding out the most effective, appropriate and feasible way of improving the quality of life of people with emphysema, for example, it is desirable to conduct a series of reviews based on specific, focused questions rather than a broad review that includes different populations, interventions and outcomes.

Systematic reviews of evidence are of significant importance when determining the best available evidence for practice. One of the most important components of this process is to have a solid protocol and search strategy in order to be able to find relevant information and produce meaningful information on which to base practice.

Significant progress has been made in recent years with regard to extending the scientific methodology and philosophies that underpin the systematic review process. A particular achievement has been the evolution of the concept of evidence, along with the broadening nature of evidence to be included in systematic reviews and thereby utilised as evidence for the facilitation of practice change. This has brought with it challenges, however, with regard to not only critical appraisal and synthesis but also the classification of evidence for recommendations. To some extent the issues surrounding the inclusion of other forms of research evidence in the systematic review process have been overcome. This being the case, the challenge becomes one of development, implementation and the auditing of clinical guidelines.

FURTHER READING

Glasziou, P., Irwig, L., Bain, C. and Colditz, G. (2001) *Systematic Reviews in Health Care*. Cambridge: Cambridge University Press.

Gough, D., Oliver, S. and Thomas, J. (eds) (2012) *An Introduction to Systematic Reviews*. London: Sage.

REFERENCES

JBI (2011) *Reviewers' Manual 2011 Edition*. The Joanna Briggs Institute, Adelaide: Australia.

Green, S., Higgins, J.P.T., Alderson, P., Clarke, M., Mulrow, C.D. and Oxman, A.D. (2008) 'Introduction', in J.P.T. Higgins, S. Green (eds), *Cochrane Handbook for Systematic Reviews of Interventions*. Chichester: John Wiley. pp. 1–6.

Jones, T. (2000) *Effectiveness of Mechanical Compression Devices in Attaining Hemostasis After Removal of a Femoral Sheath Following Femoral Artery Cannulation for Cardiac Interventional Procedures*. Adelaide: The Joanna Briggs Institute Library of Systematic Reviews.

11 Longitudinal Research

Elisabetta Ruspini with case study by
Elizabeth Mason-Whitehead

DEFINITION

'Longitudinal data' can be defined as data gathered during the observation of subjects on a number of variables over time. This definition implies the notion of repeated measurements (van der Kamp and Bijleveld, 1998). Essentially, longitudinal data present information about what happened to a set of units (people, couples, households, patient groups, firms and so on) across time. The participants in a typical longitudinal study are asked to provide information about their behaviour and attitudes regarding the issues of interest on a number of separate occasions over time (called the 'waves' of the study; Taris, 2000). In contrast, 'cross-sectional data' record the circumstances of respondents at one particular point in time. So, cross-sectional information deals with *status*, while longitudinal information concerns with *progress and change* in status.

KEY POINTS

- The focus of nursing and healthcare research is that of describing patterns of change in phenomena and evaluating the outcomes in interventions over time (Weinert, 2006)
- Most health-related phenomena of interest in nursing and healthcare science are dynamic in nature. Examples are the dynamics of well-being; individual, couple, and family coping with chronic illness; adaptation to parenthood; recovery from life-threatening and chronic illnesses

- Health is much more than the 'absence' of disease. Health is a dynamic state of well-being, the expressions of the success or failure experienced by the organism in its efforts to respond adaptively to constant environmental challenges (Bircher, 2011). For these reasons, longitudinal analysis may seem an appropriate method for health research

DISCUSSION

There are many different methods that can be used to collect longitudinal data, which means there are also many different types of research (Ruspini, 2002). The most commonly used longitudinal designs are:

- repeated cross-sectional studies carried out regularly, each time using a largely different or completely new sample (noting trends)
- prospective longitudinal studies repeatedly interview the same subjects over a period of time (panel)
- retrospective longitudinal studies (duration data) in which interviewees are asked to remember and reconstruct events and aspects of their own life courses.

Of these three, prospective studies are considered the most 'truly longitudinal' (consequently, preferable when analysing micro social change), because they periodically gather information about the same individuals (Magnusson and Bergman, 1990), asking the same sequence of questions at regular intervals.

Longitudinal data and research make it possible to:

- analyse the duration of social phenomena
- highlight differences or changes in the values of one or more variables between one period and another
- identify 'sleeper effects' – that is, connections between events and transitions that are widely separated in time because they took place in very different periods, as in the relationships between childhood, adulthood and old age – for example, the experience of old age has much to do with illness and hardship in the adult years and one's responses to these challenges as the same event or transition followed by different adaptations can lead to very different trajectories
- describe subjects' intra-individual and inter-individual changes over time and monitor the magnitude and patterns of these changes.

Longitudinal data also contribute to identifying the causes of social phenomena or at least they help to do this by allowing antecedents to be specified and consequences identified. The temporal ordering of events is often the closest we can get to causality as the structure of causality inherent in social processes may be reconstructed as a specific sequence of events leading to a certain state (Leisering and Walker, 1998). More specifically, longitudinal studies not only allow researchers to study the segment of the population that, at different points in time, finds itself caught within a specific situation, such as poverty, illness or unemployment, but also can be used in order to examine the flows into and out of such a situation, thus opening up many paths for both causal analysis and inference (Duncan, 2000).

With longitudinal data, it is also possible to develop causal theories that link individual dynamics with the dynamics of institutions and social structures – that is, they make it possible to fit the events studied into both individuals' biographies and the family and social contexts they are part of. This permits in-depth analysis of social and demographic processes in terms of both the choices and the determining factors that underlie different behaviours and situations (Gershuny, 1998).

Furthermore, the development of research projects that use longitudinal data serves to build a 'bridge' between 'quantitative' and 'qualitative' research traditions and encourages a reassessment of these concepts themselves (Holland et al., 2012; Ruspini, 1999). Within longitudinal research, great emphasis is placed on social and individual life as an interlocking series of events. This emphasis can be seen as a response to the qualitative researcher's concern to reflect the complexity of everyday life, which takes the form of a stream of interconnecting events.

Even though dynamic data offer a highly innovative and precious tool for the analysis of social phenomena, they do, nonetheless, have certain inherent disadvantages. Longitudinal research is, in itself, highly complex. It is normally more expensive, complex and time-consuming than research based on single observations. Not only do researchers have to ensure that the same subjects can be measured repeatedly over the course of many years, but they also run risks if the research team, too, cannot be preserved over the duration of the study. Consequently, longitudinal studies are usually only carried out by large research organisations and they need national and often governmental support.

CASE STUDY – ELIZABETH MASON-WHITEHEAD

Alessandro is a lecturer at a university faculty of health. He has completed a prospective longitudinal study of three years' duration. Alessandro was awarded a research grant to study undergraduate nurses through their degree programme.

The purpose of the research was to gain an understanding of the growth in professionalisation gained by students as they progressed through their courses. Alessandro wanted to know what experiences over that period of time contributed to the students' increased professionalisation. He interviewed his participants over the three years of their studies and additionally asked them to keep a diary, so they could record any instances or thoughts they may have had relating to professionalisation.

Alessandro's academic first paper from this project, entitled 'Factors affecting the growth of professionalisation in student nurses: A prospective longitudinal study', has just been published. His study produced a number of findings. One result suggested that further research is needed, particularly in relation to the role of the clinical staff, all of whom have been seen to have considerable influence on student nurses in practice.

While Alessandro found this study was time-consuming and lengthy, he appreciated that a longitudinal study was the only research method that could capture changes in experience and behaviour over a period of time. On reflection, Alessandro reported that longitudinal research is a worthwhile and rewarding experience.

CONCLUSION

In the area of nursing and healthcare research, the longitudinal form of research is essential if we want to:

- study the dynamic course of health and illness – that is, the patterns of health/illness over time for a specific individual, family, group, community and the effects of/response to multiple environmental stresses
- study the course of common diseases and their outcomes as a result of care and treatment
- analyse the impact of chronic conditions, such as arthritis, asthma, diabetes, cardiovascular diseases, and medication for these conditions, on health and health services use, chronic disease self-management and rehabilitation and the role of carers in providing services for frail aged and disabled persons
- study how (chronic) drug use patterns evolve and interact with welfare systems over time
- determine the trends in health service use within and across different population groups and communities, plus those patterns of use associated with better physical and mental health over time
- from a gender-sensitive perspective, investigate the gender dimension of health and well-being and support the gender medicine approach. The dynamic perspective can help us to improve our understanding of how women's and men's health and well-being are evolving and in what direction. Gender is an essential determinant of health and illness – data on mortality, morbidity and use of health services reveal some important differences in health experiences between women and men (see, for example, Payne, 2009). Moreover, the longitudinal approach allows us to monitor women's and men's choices, challenges and careers at crucial points during both their undergraduate and postgraduate training in health education and in their further medical careers.

FURTHER READING

Newsom, J.T., Jones, R.N. and Hofer Scott, M. (eds) (2011) *Longitudinal Data Analysis: A practical guide for researchers in aging, health, and social sciences*. New York: Routledge.
Ruspini, E. (2002) *Introduction to Longitudinal Research*. London: Routledge.

REFERENCES

Bircher, J. (2011) 'Towards a dynamic definition of health and disease', *Medicine, Health Care and Philosophy*, 8(3): 335–41. Retrieved from: http://www.ncbi.nlm.nih.gov/pubmed/16283496 (accessed 28 May 2013).
Duncan, G. (2000) 'Using panel studies to understand household behaviour and well-being', in D. Rose (ed.), *Researching Social and Economic Change: The uses of household panel studies*. Abingdon: Routledge. pp. 54–75.

Gershuny, J. (1998) 'Thinking dynamically: Sociology and narrative data', in L. Leisering and R. Walker (eds), *The Dynamics of Modern Society*. Bristol: The Policy Press. pp. 34–48.

Holland, J., Thomson, R. and Henderson, S. (2012) 'Qualitative longitudinal research: A discussion paper'. London: London South Bank University (available online at: www.lsbu.ac.uk/ahs/downloads/families/familieswp21.pdf).

Leisering, L. and Walker, R. (eds) (1998) *The Dynamics of Modern Society*. Bristol: The Policy Press.

Magnusson, D. and Bergman, L.R. (eds) (1990) *Data Quality in Longitudinal Research*. Cambridge: Cambridge University Press.

Payne, S. (2009) 'How can gender equity be addressed through health systems?', Policy Brief 12. Copenhagen: World Health Organization Regional Office for Europe, on behalf of the European Observatory on Health Systems and Policies (available online at: www.euro.who.int/__data/assets/pdf_file/0006/64941/E92846.pdf).

Ruspini, E. (ed.) (1999) 'Longitudinal analysis: A bridge between quantitative and qualitative social research', *Quality and Quantity: International Journal of Methodology* (special issue), 33 (3).

Ruspini, E. (2002) *Introduction to Longitudinal Research*. London: Routledge.

Taris, T.W. (2000) *A Primer in Longitudinal Data Analysis*. London: Sage.

van der Kamp, L.J.T. and Bijleveld, Catrien C.J.H. (1998) 'Methodological issues in longitudinal research' in C.J.H. Bijleveld et al., *Longitudinal Data Analysis: Designs, models and methods*. London: Sage. pp. 1–45.

Weinert, F.E. (2006) 'Longitudinal survey', in J.J. Fitzpatrick and M. Wallace (eds), *Encyclopaedia of Nursing Research* (2nd edn). New York: Springer. pp. 318–19.

12 Writing Research Bids

Neville J. Ford with case study by Jean Evers

DEFINITION

A research application needs to be prepared, checked carefully for accuracy, approved by the relevant institutional authorities and submitted to the funding agency. Success or failure in the process depends on the quality of the research and the proposer, how the proposal is targeted at the objectives of the funder and the competition at that particular time.

KEY POINTS

The following 12 stages in the process of preparing applications are proposed. Each of the following steps is important and, if followed carefully, can reduce the likelihood of wasted effort:

1. defining the research project
2. selecting a funding body
3. deciding when to apply
4. forming the team
5. formulating the proposal
6. aligning with the funders' objectives
7. the critical friend
8. costings and authorisation
9. demand management
10. managing adventure and risk
11. submitting the proposal
12. dealing with peer review

DISCUSSION

Defining the research project

The first stage is to establish a clear understanding of the research project under consideration. Funders like to see a definite and specific statement of research objectives and questions that will be answered. It needs to set out how the research is likely to provide useful outcomes that are worth funding. Careful consideration of the scope and limitations of the project enable the applicant to write a convincing argument for the funder about why the proposal is likely to provide value for money. In the author's experience, many applicants write their detailed proposals far too early and before the key research questions have been established.

Selecting a funding body

There are many bodies that fund research, from the world-famous national and international funding agencies, such as the UK research councils, to major charities funding specific areas of work, to local charities and trusts that may be able to support work in their localities.

Common to all these potential sources of funding is an excessive number of applications and a consequent need for funders to have a selection process that ensures funded projects meets their funders' objectives. Researchers applying for funding often do little research into the funding bodies' objectives and reasons for providing the funding, so do not always provide the required evidence that their proposal fully meets the funder's objectives.

Funders operate in two main modes. The simplest is the 'call for proposals'. Typically, such a call will be issued and given a specific timeframe, with details of the application process, the deadline and provide a clear indication of the type of project that the funder is looking to support.

The second mode is known as the 'responsive mode'. Here, funders welcome applications from people who have good ideas and respond to the ideas generated. With this mode, there may still be a deadline, there is likely to be specific guidance on the form applications should take and there will be some details of any restrictions on what may be considered. It is tempting to think that this mode provides researchers with greater freedom to propose a project of a particular type, but, in practice, both modes are highly competitive. With the responsive mode there is a need to first capture the interest of the funder in a particular type of project that might have been self-evident in a more focused call.

Apart from the mode of funding proposals, funding bodies also have a range of objectives and applications need to align with these if they are to be successful. Is the funder primarily concerned with training researchers, supporting world-class research, developing infrastructure and intellectual property (IP) that will support future commercial work or providing answers to key health questions? Divining this information will help to indicate both the types of teams and the types of projects that the funder is likely to support.

Researchers are often heard to say, They can only say 'No' when they try to apply to a funder for a project that does not meet its requirements. With experience, researchers come to realise that 'No' is precisely the response that they will get in this case and their time and effort may well have been wasted and there may well also be some reputational damage from making a poor or ill-focused application.

Deciding when to apply

Research funders expect projects to be of a high quality, answer suitable research questions, low risk and timely. These are the guiding principles for when to submit an application. Most funders who publish deadlines will be happy to confirm future likely deadlines for similar competitions and, indeed, putting an application off until a later deadline may often be the best way to ensure that it is focused, based on a clear assessment of the current state of the art and has taken all possible steps to limit risk to the project.

Forming the team

The implementation of any research project is an important issue for funders and is often dealt with less than adequately in proposals. The key questions to answer in forming the team are as follows.

Where?

Presumably the applicant has a clear idea about where the project will be undertaken, but the funder needs to be convinced that this is a suitable location. Sometimes there is a need for specialist facilities and to interact with other researchers or specialisms. So, the task is to explain why this location is the right one. Sometimes that will be easy, but, on other occasions, researchers may reflect that there is a centre elsewhere that would be a more natural place to undertake the work. If this is the case, then there is a risk that the funder will not consider the project to be good value, simply because of the choice of host. Sometimes forming some sort of collaboration with the 'obvious' centre can mitigate the risk of the proposal being rejected.

Who?

It may be obvious to applicants that this is their project and they should be lead researchers or principal investigators (PI). This may not be so clear to the potential funder, however, especially where the applicants have little previous experience as PIs. Here, the formation of a suitable research team, including experienced leaders, reasonably independent people as members of a steering or management group and all those who will conduct the work, is the best approach. A suitable team should demonstrate a balance between experience, specific research knowledge, independence and objectivity.

Why and how?

The final elements in putting together the research team are based on considering who the beneficiaries of the research will be (in other words, *why* the research is appropriate) and who will need to collaborate in order to provide access to the data subjects and so on (*how* the project will actually happen). Involving these people as members of the team or steering group will demonstrate to funders that applicants have thought about how to maximise the impact and minimise the risks associated with the project.

Formulating the proposal

Funding bodies look for answers to a range of questions and it is tempting to focus on the obvious ones, such as why this is a valuable research project and why the research team has the right people to do the work.

Typically, proposals need to demonstrate familiarity with the current state of the art in the field, an understanding of appropriate research objectives and questions, an appropriate methodology and a research team with access to the facilities required to undertake the work, as well as clear plans to disseminate the outcomes and linkages with potential users of the work. The work plan needs to take account of likely risks and contingencies and demonstrate how the project will be monitored and managed by people who have sufficient independence and objectivity to point out when mistakes are made.

Common mistakes in preparing proposals include a lack of focus on specifying the research objectives and the likely value of the research outcomes, poor work plans, a failure to justify the budget and explain the facilities available to undertake the work, as well as a lack of understanding of risk.

Aligning with the funders' objectives

Once the first draft of a proposal is available, it is necessary to revisit the funders' criteria, to check that the original plans have not changed so the project will no longer be of interest to the funders. Check once more that the funders really want to fund this type of project and make sure the application highlights the ways in which the proposal meets the funders' own agenda. Try to be explicit and specific about this. Many proposals fail to demonstrate to the funders why the researchers should be funded from the scarce funds available for the particular scheme.

The critical friend

Try to find somebody with experience of grant-awarding committees who will read your applications critically. It is common for the authors of proposals to have missed something obvious that poses a major risk to the project and could be addressed before sending them in. Applicants need advice from somebody who is prepared to tell them what these omissions are and thank them later for their (often unwelcome) advice. Fixing these more obvious flaws can more than double the chances of success, so this is a key stage, but one frequently missed out.

Costings and authorisation

It is safe to assume the organisation that will host the project will have its own governance and authorisation rules it follows before a proposal is submitted. It is important to investigate early on what the timescales will be for this authorisation because missed internal deadlines may mean that an excellent application cannot be submitted in time. Usually, part of the authorisation should be given very early in the process, based on a draft version of the proposal, with the final authorisation speeded up because the initial work has been done early. This is the point at which costings, overhead rates, internal requirements for ethical review and the appointment of any staff will be considered and authorised. Without institutional support, the project will not be able to happen.

Demand management

A recent introduction by many major funders is the requirement for institutions to undertake demand management procedures to reduce the number of fair, good and very good proposals that are submitted at all because they are not excellent. Applicants need to be aware that their proposals are increasingly likely to need to go through this stage, which may extend time delays between the application being ready to submit and the institution being able to submit it.

Managing adventure and risk

Major funding agencies talk about supporting *adventurous* research (which is good), but they will not fund high-risk research. A key part of the application process is demonstrating that the research objectives are exciting and adventurous, but risks have been mitigated by appropriate management and contingency planning.

Submitting the proposal

Most proposals are submitted using an online submission system, which makes things quick, but not always simple. Make sure to allow time to learn how to register on the system, upload the application and for any local submission or authorisation to take place in advance of the deadline. For paper-based applications, it is important to have an independent second check that all the documents (including multiple copies) actually go into the envelope. Sending by courier rather than standard post is the norm.

For both electronic and postal submissions, funding bodies complain that around one third of applications received are incomplete. Read your application and the guidelines carefully – are letters of support, copies of CVs or other supporting documents required?

Dealing with peer review

Usually, after a delay of three to six months, applicants receive details of the peer review comments. These may be in advance of the meeting that will discuss the project or afterwards, as part of the feedback process. Whether the project will be funded or not, this is a chance to learn from the feedback how to write a better application next time. Sometimes, there is a chance to submit corrections to factual errors in the review reports, but this is not an opportunity to rewrite the proposal and make further representations. Occasionally, resubmission of a rejected proposal may be encouraged, but the best advice is usually to learn from the feedback and start with a new proposal that builds on the lessons learnt.

CASE STUDY – JEAN EVERS

Ali is a senior lecturer in public health nursing and recently achieved accreditation as a fellow with the Higher Education Academy (HEA). Julie is a senior teaching fellow at the Faculty of Health and Social Care and is keen to support and develop Ali's research potential. Following Ali's successful accreditation, Julie found an opportunity with the HEA that would be beneficial for Ali's professional development. Ali had a potential research project she had been considering for some time and had discussed with Julie. Following discussions with practice partners and changes in government policy, it become evident that there was a need for research in public health nursing.

Following the initial meeting with Julie, Ali felt overwhelmed as the principal investigator. She had difficulty understanding the HEA's criteria, objectives and specific requirements, particularly how she was to get it all done by the required deadline. Julie shared examples of her previous funding applications, which enabled Ali to progress and develop a detailed research proposal that aligned with the HEA guidelines. Ali also found it challenging mapping the research proposal to the required theme to attract the HEA funding, but Julie was able to direct Ali to their previous discussions, explaining how the research could embrace the required theme. Julie also recommended collecting additional data that had the potential to enhance the research findings.

Ali met Julie to peer review the draft proposal and discuss the project costings. This meeting was also to ensure that the required institutional authorisation and governance arrangements were completed. If the university's requirements were not adhered to the project would not be able to progress, even if the funding was granted. Julie embraced her role as a critical friend by supporting and signposting Ali throughout the process. As Julie was an HEA reviewer, this was advantageous to Ali's success with the grant submission. The university research office also supported Ali through the grant submission process.

Ali successfully won the grant, having gained confidence in writing grant applications and developing research proposals. Ali was also supported by Julie throughout the research in relation to its implementation, writing progress reports and managing the budget. The ongoing support from this critical friend was an important component in the overall success of the project.

CONCLUSION

Researchers will spend a considerable proportion of their careers writing grant applications and designing project proposals. Even the most successful are unlikely to be funded more than one quarter of the time, so it is important to learn how to focus time and effort on the most likely positive outcomes and learn from the feedback about failures. Hopefully, by choosing the right funder for a particular project proposal, putting the right team together and getting as much feedback as possible before submitting the proposal, the chances of success when making such applications will be as high as possible.

FURTHER READING

Beins, B.C. (2012) *Successful Research Projects: A step-by-step guide*. London: Sage.

Bell, J. (2010) *Doing Your Research Project: A guide for first-time researchers in education, health and social science* (5th edn). Maidenhead: Open University Press and McGraw-Hill.

Denscombe, M. (2012) *Research Proposals: A practical guide*. Maidenhead: Open University Press, McGraw-Hill.

Part 2

Qualitative Research Methods

Chris Whitney-Cooper

DEFINITION

'Action research' is an approach to research that uses a cyclical process of problem-solving by identifying and implementing actions to solve those problems with participants (Reason and Bradbury, 2007). The strength of action research is its ability to influence practice (action) while simultaneously gathering data to share with a wider audience (inquiry) (Stringer, 2007). In contrast to conventional social science, the primary purpose of action research is to not just understand social situations but also effect a desired change to generate knowledge and empower participants (Reason and Torbert, 2001).

Reason and Bradbury (2007: 1) suggested that defining action research is problematic because it is a 'family of practices of living inquiry that aims, in a great variety of ways, to link practice and ideas in the service of human flourishing. It is not so much a methodology as an orientation to inquiry that seeks to create participative communities of inquiry'. This suggests that action research is more of an orientation to research than a discrete methodology sharing a number of key characteristics.

KEY POINTS

- Action research is enacted by means of an iterative action–inquiry cycle
- There are three important elements:
  - participation
  - action
  - the simultaneous contribution to knowledge and change.
- The researcher needs to be immersed in the research setting, working *with* participants to facilitate the development of an authentic (valid) narrative that comes from the participants
- Validity and rigour are achieved by means of the conscious and deliberate enactment of the action research cycle
- There are unique ethical considerations due to the dynamic and iterative nature of action research

DISCUSSION

The action–inquiry cycle

Action research is a cyclical problem-solving process of identifying a problem and implementing a way of solving it (Stringer, 2007). The research is rooted in the social psychology of action emerging from social interaction and 'learning by doing' (Pedler, 2011). A core concept of this intellectual and practical engagement is 'praxis', as (Noffke and Stevenson 1995: 1):

> critical thought and the continuous interplay of doing something and revising our thoughts about what ought to be done.

Praxis creates a kind of 'cultural interruption', resulting in those involved reconsidering their behaviour, implementing actions based on their understanding and, in so doing, creating change. Knowledge arises in the context of practice that is meaningful to the participants, so researchers need to work *with* participants (Huang, 2010). This typically involves creating spaces in which researchers and participants engage together in cycles of action and critical reflection (Reason and McArdle, 2008).

The iterative action–inquiry cycle (see Figure 13.1) breaks down into four phases:

- **diagnosing** – identifying the problem
- **planning** – exploring how to solve the problem
- **implementing** – putting the agreed solutions into action
- **evaluating** – seeing if the actions were successful.

The fourth phase then feeds back into the first, diagnosing, phase. A variety of researchers have abbreviated and/or expanded the descriptions of these phases, but essentially the process remains the same.

An action research study can go through several of these cycles. The repeated cycles are sometimes depicted as a spiral model as the cycles build on each other to create a transformative change. It is important to note that Figure 13.1 and

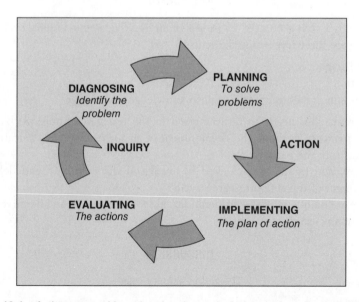

Figure 13.1 Action research's action–inquiry cycle (adapted from Baskerville, 1999)

other models are two-dimensional representations of a three-dimensional practice so they can create an image of events moving through a linear process, whereas the reality is more complex. During each cycle, participants can repeat processes, revise procedures, rethink interpretations, sometimes 'leapfrog' phases and make radical changes in direction (Stringer, 2007). Action research is, by nature, an iterative process and such growth is at the heart of 'good' action research. As Reason and Bradbury (2007: 2) suggest:

> good action research emerges over time in an evolutionary and developmental process, as individuals develop skills of inquiry and as communities of inquiry develop within communities of practice.

Participation, action and change

The methodologies of action research have shifted over time, developing out of a range of approaches within a quantitative scientific approach, then moving towards social change and a more qualitative and social constructivist methodology (Hart and Bond, 1995). 'Qualitative action research', therefore, can draw on interpretative or critical approaches to understand reality that affects the nature of participation, change and knowledge. Similarly, critical theory has been extended in some qualitative research approaches, called 'participatory action research' (Reason and Bradbury 2007), as a way of enabling participants to change a power imbalance. All approaches, however, centre on (Carr and Kemmis, 1986):

- **participation** – the nature of the democratic impulse
- **action** – the change intervention
- **knowledge and change** – the simultaneous contribution to social science.

Participation

The egalitarian principle of qualitative action research is that participants are 'active', in contrast to the passive nature of the 'subjects' of traditional research. An important element of participation is how people are drawn into and collaborate in the processes of the inquiry and action. The degree of democratic participation (empowerment and equality) in action research depends on the philosophical position of the researchers and the assumptions of the ontology on which they draw.

Participation is not neutral and can be influenced by the nature of the relationship with the researchers and or organisations involved, thus affecting the validity of the findings (Coghlan and Brannick, 2005). The aim is to achieve as high a level of participation as possible.

Action, knowledge and change

Action research has at its core change. That change can be a practical issue, theory generation or an evaluation of an innovation (Stringer, 2007). Not all projects implement a change as part of the cyclical process, particularly if the outcome is deemed to be not feasible or unacceptable. This still constitutes action research even though the intervention is not accepted, as the participants will have learned something new and, in the process, change has occurred in their understanding, beliefs, values and/or behaviour (Reason and Bradbury, 2007).

The role of the researchers

All research requires willing subjects, but the collaborative partnership between the 'researchers' and 'researched' in an action research study means the demarcation between the two may not be evident. Action researchers need to be immersed in the research to negotiate the actions and the interpretation of that journey between all the different parties involved. Whether the researchers are 'insiders' or 'outsiders' they can inhabit both roles at different points in the study enabling their project to have authenticity (Coghlan and Brannick, 2005). Action researchers must work *with* practitioners and aim to report the construction of a 'group narrative' (Winter, 2002) in order to create an authentic (valid) story from the participants' perspectives.

Validity and rigour

Discussions about validity in qualitative action research mirror the debates in the wider qualitative research literature concerning the meaning of validity in a 'post-positivist' context and the nature of reality (Waterman, 1995).

Qualitative action research has been criticised for not being 'valid' as the data collected is highly specific and not generalisable. Reason and Bradbury (2007) argue that action research should not 'mimic' other research types as its validity comes from the transparent articulation of an emerging consensus of understanding. Rigour is achieved by the transparency with which the data are generated and how events are questioned and interpreted in multiple action research cycles.

The broad processes to improve validity include (Stringer, 2007):

- **triangulation** – assessing data from different sources
- **quality of observations** – achieved by prolonged and persistent observations in the field
- **practical utility** – ensuring the emerging concepts and constructions are adequate to account for the phenomena investigated
- **participatory validity** – obtaining participant and peer confirmation.

Ethical issues

The same ethical principles apply to action research as any other form of research (respect for participants, prevention of harm, assurance of confidentiality or anonymity and maintenance of privacy), but the relationships between researchers and participants raise some unique ethical issues in relation to anonymity, confidentiality and consent.

Anonymity and confidentiality

An action research study can jeopardise the possibility of confidentiality and anonymity as the participants know each other (Waterman, 1995). This creates confusion about what can be shared during the project and when publishing the final report. These difficulties can be addressed by creating ground rules regarding what can or cannot be shared by gaining agreement from participants as to the ways in which information is presented.

Consent

The mixed roles that action researchers can inhabit (researcher, co-worker, participant) can create ambiguous lines of communication, leading to situations in which it may be difficult to gain 'genuine' consent. The dynamic, iterative nature of action research means that full informed consent may not be possible when the nature of the proposed change is unknown and participants don't know what they are consenting to. This only becomes an issue, however, if gaining consent is seen as a single event rather than reviewing and renegotiating consent within the cyclical process.

CASE STUDY

Action research is useful for organisational change and innovation. A project was used to research capacity building within the workforce in an NHS trust (Moore et al., 2011). The critical action research project was managed by three researchers employed by the trust, two outsiders and one insider. The insider enabled immersion within the organisation's culture in order to identify key people (16) to be part of the project's steering group.

The project's stages and findings

- **Diagnosing** – Achieved via semi-structured interviews. They identified innovation to research, but also that there was no infrastructure to support the research.
- **Planning** – An action plan was developed to put an infrastructure in place.
- **Implementing** – The action plan was managed to create an infrastructure and support for identified innovators in the trust who could change the culture.
- **Evaluating** – This phase recognised that the research was not embedded in the culture, so the project was funded for further development cycles in order to implement the research strategy.

There was practical utility as the findings reflected the views of the participants. Participation validity was achieved by involving the participants in the steering group and sharing the findings with the staff in the trust.

Ethical approval was achieved via the local research ethics committee, although it was acknowledged that authentic relationships between the action researchers and the participants in the research were central to ensuring that ethical consent would continue to be given.

CONCLUSION

Action research is a particular orientation towards doing research rather than a discrete methodology in its own right. It is a participative and iterative change process using an action–inquiry cycle. Validity is achieved by means of the participation of those being researched, rather than them being 'subjects', and the conscious negotiated implementation of the cycle to develop an authentic account of the research journey.

Action research is particularly suited to identifying problems and developing potential solutions to improve organisational and clinical practice.

FURTHER READING

Coghlan, D. and Brannick, T. (2005) *Doing Action Research in your own Organisation* (2nd edn). London: Sage.

Stringer, E.T. (2007) *Action Research: A handbook for practitioners* (3rd edn). Thousand Oaks, CA: Sage.

REFERENCES

Baskerville (1999) 'Investigating information systems with action research', *Communications of the Association of Information systems*, 2 (19) (available online, if you have permission, at: ftp://ftp.cba.uri.edu/classes/N_Dholakia/URI-MKT697Q/Baskerville-IS-Action-Research.pdf).

Carr, W. and Kemmis, S. (1986) *Becoming Critical: Education, knowledge and action research*. Victoria, Australia: Deakin University Press.

Coghlan, D. and Brannick, T. (2005) *Doing Action Research in Your Own Organisation* (2nd edn). London: Sage.

Hart, E. and Bond, M. (1995) *Action Research for Health and Social Care: A guide to practice*. Buckingham: Open University Press.

Huang, H.M. (2010) 'What is good action research?: Why the resurgent interest?', *Action Research*, 8: 93.

Moore, J., Crozier, K. and Kite, K. (2011) 'An action research approach for developing research and innovation in nursing and midwifery practice: Building research capacity in one NHS foundation trust'. *Nurse Education Today*, 32: 39–45.

Noffke, S. and Stevenson, R.B. (1995) *Educational Action Research: Becoming practically critical*. New York and London: Teachers College Press.

Pedler, M. (2011) *Action Research in Practice* (4th edn). Farnham: Gower.

Reason, P. and Bradbury, H. (2007) *The Handbook of Action Research* (2nd edn). London: Sage.

Reason, P. and McArdle, M. (2008) 'Action research and organization development', in T.C. Cummings (ed.), *Handbook of Organization Development*. London: Sage. pp. 123–36.

Reason, P. and Torbert, W. (2001) 'The action turn: Toward a transformational social science', *Concepts and Transformation*, 6 (1): 1–37.

Stringer, E.T. (2007) *Action Research: A handbook for practitioners* (3rd edn). Thousand Oaks, CA: Sage.

Waterman H. (1995) 'Distinguishing between "traditional" and action research', *Nurse Researcher*, 2 (3): 15–23.

Winter, R. (2002) 'Truth or fiction: Problems of validity and authenticity in narratives of action research', *Educational Action Research*, 10 (1): 143–54.

key concepts in nursing and healthcare research

Andy Lovell

DEFINITION

'Case study research' varies according to the 'unit of analysis', which, in sociology, might be the social group (family, ethnic group, community), in psychology, the individual, for the economist, the firm, and the political scientist, the nation state, region or electoral system (Gerring, 2007). The case study, irrespective of which unit is selected, relies implicitly on the establishment of a micro–macro association in social behaviour (Alexander et al., 1987).

Case study research, in the context of healthcare, might be utilised as a means of studying issues such as patient experience, staff culture or systemic change in order to analyse wider concerns within the healthcare system.

KEY POINTS

- Case study research focuses on one unit of analysis, such as a group of individuals with a shared issue for study, and contextualises this according to the prevailing conditions
- Multiple methods of data collection are employed, particularly, though not exclusively, qualitative, as well as individual interviews, focus groups, participant and non-participant observations and documentary material
- Naturalistic generalisation suggests that skilled case study researchers enhance their understanding and appreciation of a situation via their experience of undertaking research in previous situations
- The classic case study revolves around an individual's relationship with a specific phenomenon, such as being diagnosed as terminally ill, in the context of the family, community, institution or wider social structures

DISCUSSION

Background

Case study research involves 'study of the singular, the particular, the unique' (Simons, 2009: 3), has a long history in a range of disciplines, such as sociology, social anthropology, psychology and education, and primarily, though not exclusively (see Yin, 2009, for example), focuses on qualitative data collection methods, such as open-ended interviews, participant observation and archive or documentary analysis. It seeks in-depth study of the case(s) by means of detailed investigation of a specific area of interest or phenomenon and sets out to 'locate the global in the local', the careful selection of the research site being the most crucial element in the analytic process (Hamel et al., 1993: 38).

The case study methodology is particularly useful for answering 'How?' or 'Why?' questions, allows investigators little control over events and concentrates on a contemporary phenomenon within a real-life context (Yin, 2009). It is particularly, though not exclusively, suited to the work of qualitative researchers, embodying, perhaps, the three key word characteristic of any qualitative method: describing, understanding and explaining (Granger, 1988).

A phenomenon that might be chosen for a study in relation to healthcare, for example, could be one from a range of issues as diverse as interpersonal violence, organisational restructuring or the experience of illness. The emphasis in any such study is on clear and considered description of the phenomenon by means of a process of 'totalizing in the observation, reconstruction and analysis of the objects under study' (Zonabend, 1992: 52). An in-depth exploration of the experience of self-injury, for example, is likely to benefit from unstructured interviews with self-injurers, more structured interviews with significant others and analysis of documents. It should, therefore, be tentatively linked to the relationship between the individual self-injurer and society.

Case study research should be informed by theory – specifically, how the researcher's worldview is reflected in the construction, implementation, progress and subsequent evaluation of the study. Many contemporary qualitative researchers, for example, adopt a position of the world being a construction, an anti-essentialist position wherein there exist multiple truths and no single universal reality (Stake, 1995). Social constructionist thinking, however, constitutes only *one* theoretical approach and there are many other positions, arising from a range of disciplines, that might inform any research project.

The classic case study surrounds the life story of the individual or group and shows how this throws light on a specific phenomenon, such as that person's or group's experience of mental health services or cancer. It has its roots in the Chicago School of Sociology in the 1930s and traditionally concentrates on outsiders' life experience on the periphery of society (see Bennett, 1981, for a comprehensive history).

Key principles

Prior to undertaking any data collection, how the voluminous case study data will be analysed needs to be given comprehensive consideration. Making it manageable may involve the construction of matrices of categories, systems of flowcharts, cross-tabulations of frequencies (Miles and Huberman, 1984), pattern matching, explanation-building and time-series analysis (Yin, 2009). The purpose of the research, however, should guide the choice of analysis methods and systems. Plummer (2001: 153) points out that 'insights, understanding, appreciation, intimate familiarity are the goals and not "facts", explanations or generalizations'. There is, nevertheless, a commitment to avoiding the possibility of criticisms of sloppiness, perfunctoriness, incompetence, corruption and dishonesty identified by Bromley (1986: xiii), while remaining true to the story.

One particularly useful analytical tool frequently favoured by case study researchers is a solidly structured thematic analysis, as advocated by the likes of Burnard (1991) and Braun and Clarke (2006). A structured thematic analysis provides the various stages requisite for an approach to analysis whereby the data are worked, reworked, codes and categories identified and subsequently organised into strong themes.

There is a requirement on the part of case study researchers to specify the criteria by which their work should be judged. This is particularly true of the thorny issue of generalisation, some arguing for its redundancy in qualitative approaches and others that there needs to be some wider significance.

'Naturalistic generalisation' is most associated with the work of Stake (1995: 5), who argues that the most important skills for researchers studying human affairs are 'the natural powers of people to experience and understand'. He (1995: 6) goes on to consider how naturalistic generalisations develop within a person as a consequence of experience, emphasise expectation, not prediction, and 'derive from the tacit knowledge of how things are, why they are, how people feel about them, and how these things are likely to be later or in other places with which this person is familiar'.

The main concern, nevertheless, is ensuring that case study research is rigorous, exerts its considerable strengths of theoretical validation, strategic approach to analysis and insights into the human condition. It must be ethically sound in its purpose, robustly constructed and interpreted creatively yet with full integrity.

Critique and response

Critics of case study research have emphasised the risk of excessive and sometimes unnecessary data collection, the 'error of misplaced precision' and the intrinsic superiority of experimental research (Campbell and Stanley, 1963). One of these authors, however, subsequently acknowledged that case study design should be judged according to the criteria set out (Cook and Campbell, 1979). Other writers suggest that the intrinsic hardness of the experimental method is misguided and ask if complete objectivity can ever be achievable and consider the concept of 'scientific knowledge' dubious (Chalmers, 1982). In effect, methodological concerns are unlikely to be resolved by qualitative/quantitative tension (Hamel et al., 1993) and the perpetuation of 'failed debates' (Pires, 1982).

CASE STUDY

In healthcare, the case study method is especially worthy of consideration for the investigation of individual lives linked together by experiencing a particular phenomenon.

Lovell (2007), for example, examined the life stories of 15 people with learning disabilities, all having a history of engaging in self-injury stretching back over many years. Self-injury and the process by which it became entrenched in these people's lives constituted the phenomenon under investigation, the individual life stories the specific cases for analysis. Those in this group were bound by their propensity for self-injury, experiences of health and other services and difficulties with verbal communication, yet separated by their life circumstances and particular experiences of causing themselves damage.

A social constructionist stance was adopted in order to accentuate the fact that self-injury may vary according to time and space and if we define it according to biological or psychological criteria, then we are likely to treat it according to such criteria.

The study required the construction of chronological case histories detailing the emergence and consolidation of self-injury over the course of the people's early lives as their ages ranged from 18 to 45 years. Data collection consisted a series of semi-structured interviews with parents and significant others, the examination of documents, such as clinical notes, professional reports and personal correspondence, and periods of non-participant observation. The majority of the group (nine) lived in their family homes, the remainder (six) living in residential accommodation.

The multiple sources for the data collection inherent within the case study method helped to facilitate its being sociologically informed research, suggesting, for example, that greater exploration of the social context surrounding an individual's self-injury might extend and perhaps challenge the currently dominant biological and psychological perspectives. The study laid emphasis on the process by which people engage with self-injury over time and put forward the concept of a 'career' (following Goffman, 1961) as a means of enhancing our understanding of the complex relationship between individuals and self-injury.

CONCLUSION

Case study research has a long history, was once the method of choice for many researchers and, at the time of writing, is enjoying something of a revival. Its main strengths relate to the amount of data generated and the considerable diversity of collection methods employed, though the key to them resides in thorough and informed analysis.

Qualitative methods frequently make more sense to healthcare workers than quantitative ones as they fit well with their interest in people usually having guided their choice of career. Also, case studies are the most pertinent approach when studying individual experiences, serving, as they do, to contextualise life stories in terms of vicissitudes such as social, political and economic conditions.

The role of the researchers is crucial in bearing witness to people's stories, informing their perceptions and insights with theoretical considerations. People with learning disabilities, mental health difficulties, the elderly and other groups susceptible to stigmatisation are particularly significant in case study work – the legacy of the Chicago School of Sociology, perhaps – as it provides a lens through which to view the lives of vulnerable individuals and a means of interpreting their experience. According to Butterfield (1951: 6), however, 'the only understanding we ever reach in history is but a refinement, more or less subtle and sensitive, of the difficult – and sometimes deceptive – process of imagining oneself in another person's place'.

FURTHER READING

Plummer, K. (2001) *Documents of Life 2: An invitation to critical humanism*. London: Sage.
Thomas, W.I. and Znaniecka, F. (Zaretsky, E., ed.) (1996) *The Polish Peasant in Europe and America: A classic work in immigration history*. Chicago, IL: University of Illinois Press.

REFERENCES.

Alexander, J., Giesen, B., Munch, R. and Smelser, N. (eds) (1987) *The Micro–Macro Link*. Berkeley, CA: University of California Press.
Bennett, J. (1981) *Oral History and Delinquency: The rhetoric of criminology*. Chicago, IL: University of Chicago Press.
Braun, V. and Clarke, V. (2006) 'Using thematic analysis in psychology', *Qualitative Research in Psychology*, 3: 77–101.
Bromley, D. (1986) *The Case Study Method in Psychology and Related Disciplines*. Chichester: Wiley.
Burnard, P. (1991) 'A method of analysing interview transcripts in qualitative research', *Nurse Education Today*, 11: 461–66.
Butterfield, H. (1951) *History and Human Relations*. London: Collins.
Campbell, D.T. and Stanley, J.C. (1963) 'Experimental and quasi-experimental designs for research on teaching', in N.L. Cage (ed.), *Handbook of Research and Teaching*. Chicago, IL: Rand McNally. pp. 13–25.
Chalmers, A.F. (1982) *What is This Thing Called Science* (2nd edn). Buckingham: Open University Press.
Cook, T.D. and Campbell, D.T. (1979) *Quasi-experimentation: Design and analysis issues for field settings*. Boston, MA: Houghton Mifflin.
Gerring, J. (2007) *Case Study Research: Principles and practices*. Cambridge: Cambridge University Press.
Goffman, E. (1961) *Asylums: Essays on the social situation of mental patients and other inmates*. Harmondsworth: Penguin.
Granger, G.-G. (1988) *Pour la Connaissance Philosophique* [For philosophical knowledge]. Paris: Odile Jacob.
Hamel, J., Dufour, S. and Fortin, J. (1993) *Case Study Methods: Qualitative Research Methods Series 32*. London: Sage.
Lovell, A. (2007) 'Learning disability against itself: The self-injury/self-harm conundrum', *British Journal of Learning Disabilities*, 36: 109–21.
Miles, M. and Huberman, M. (1984) *Qualitative Data Analysis: A source book for new methods*. Thousand Oaks, CA: Sage.
Pires, A.P. (1982) 'Qualitative method in North America: A debate that failed (1918–1960)', *Sociological Society*, 14 (1): 15–29.
Plummer, K. (2001) *Documents of Life 2: An invitation to critical humanism*. London: Sage.
Simons, H. (2009) *Case Study Research in Practice*. London: Sage.
Stake, R.E. (1995) *The Art of Case Study Research*. London: Sage.
Yin, R.K. (2009) *Case Study Research: Design and methods*. London: Sage.
Zonabend, F. (1992) 'The monograph in European ethnology', *Current Sociology*, 40 (1): 49–54.

15   Ethnography

Annette McIntosh-Scott with case study by
Jenni Templeman

DEFINITION

'Ethnography' is the art and science of describing a group or society in relation to their culture, customs, habits and differences. It involves exploration of the group in a bid to understand, discover, describe and interpret a way of life from the point of view of its participants.

Ethnography is based on a phenomenologically orientated paradigm that embraces a multicultural perspective and acknowledges that there are multiple realities (O'Leary 2004; Robson, 2011). The term 'ethnography' can both describe the research methodology and be applied to the finished descriptive account (Bryman, 2012).

KEY POINTS

- Ethnography is qualitative in nature and uses a variety of research methods, normally incorporating observation
- The advantages of ethnography include the insights and understanding generated from a group and consequent emerging theories
- Ethnography has challenges that have to be recognised, anticipated and acknowledged
- Ethnography can be a valuable research method for use within health and social care

DISCUSSION

Ethnography is built on the belief that individuals process the world with reference to cultural experience, both in terms of constructs and constraints, and explores methods, rules, roles and expectations that structure any particular situation (O'Leary, 2004; Fetterman, 1998).

Ethnography derived from anthropology and traditionally required the total immersion of researchers in a community or society so that a detailed account of the life and culture of the group could be developed. The term 'thick description' was coined by Geertz (1973) to encapsulate the rich accounts coming out of such research.

78

Originally, ethnography focused on exotic cultures, but it has evolved to become widely used as a contemporary social research method in which the focus of the research is the uncovering of sociocultural meanings in communities or groups (Robson, 2011). Ethnography is therefore generally concerned with exploring concepts, producing description and developing explanations or theories (Hammersley and Atkinson, 2007).

There are various forms of ethnography including:

- traditional
- interpretative, which draws on experiential knowledge
- critical, in which the description is informed by socialist and/or feminist politics
- advocate (Fetterman, 1998)/practical (Brewer, 2000), in which participants define their reality and the ideal solution to their problems and the researchers take an active role in bringing about change
- auto ethnography.

There is no specific design for an ethnographic study – depth rather than breadth is the general aim, with small sample sizes, description and interpretation being the norm (Robson, 2011).

Data collection and analysis

Traditionally, ethnography involved researchers participating in extensive fieldwork or observation of the groups in question. This was to gain an 'emic perspective', which is one that comes from the insider's point of view, in contrast to an 'etic perspective', which is an outsider's viewpoint. Today, too, in ethnography researchers strive to uncover the emic view and 'tacit knowledge' – that is, information so ingrained groups are not conscious of it (Polit and Hungler, 1999).

Robson (2011) thought observation could be either formal and structured or informal and less structured and that the choice of approach is often guided by the research questions. This, in turn, guides the gathering and recording of information. The ethnographic approach usually combines a number of methods, although a dominant one may be used (Hammersley and Atkinson, 2007), including the following.

- **Observation** – The roles adopted by the researchers determines the extent of their participation in the research situation and can range from complete observers, who use an observation measurement instrument of some kind, and complete participants, who, as Robson (2011) notes, are the instruments. Bryman (2012) outlines six roles researchers can assume.

  o **Covert full member** – This involves researchers concealing their true role and striving to become members of the communities they are studying. This is rare to find in contemporary research studies as the deception involved can be hard to justify.

- o **Overt full member** – Where the researchers are full members of the groups and their status is known.
- o **Participating observer** – Where the researchers are not full members of the groups being studied, but undertake shared activities.
- o **Partially participating observer** – This role mirrors that of the above, but observation is not always the main method of collecting data – more use is made of interviews or document analysis.
- o **Minimally participating observer** – As the name suggests, the researchers undertake observation, but interact only in a minimal way with the groups they are studying.
- o **Non-participating observer** – In this role, the researchers take no part in the group's activities and generally interact via interviews.

- **Field notes** – These supplement and enrich the data and add to the thick description of the studies.
- **Interviews/informal discussions** – These can either be unstructured – especially, as Hammersley and Atkinson (2007) noted, at the beginning of the research – or follow a more structured format.
- **Document analysis**.
- **Reflexive diary or notes** – These include elements such as personal reflections and feelings and help contextualise and document the effects of researchers on the process.

Additionally, as Bryman (2012) stated, there has been an increase in the use of visual materials and online methods in research, including ethnography. Fetterman (1998) and Robson (2011) noted that, in many applied settings, long-term continuous fieldwork is neither desirable nor possible and, often, it is feasible only to apply ethnographic techniques to the *area* of study rather than undertake a full-blown ethnography. Wolcott (1999) opined that some ethnographically based studies rely almost exclusively on interviews, especially where participant observation is not a realistic option.

The analysis of data is not undertaken in relation to a set structure. As Hammersley and Atkinson (2007: 158) state, 'it is important to recognise that there is no formula or recipe for the analysis of ethnographic data'. Readers are directed to their chapter on the process of analysis for further guidance.

Strengths of ethnography

O'Leary (2004) considered that the strengths of ethnography include offering ways to explore the working nature and norms of a culture, leading to a dialogue with existing theories as well as insights, which, in turn, can generate more theories. It also offers an approach for generating understandings from the perspectives of the researched.

Hammersley and Atkinson (2007) noted that a virtue of ethnography is its flexibility and responsiveness to the local setting and context. Robson (2011) stated that one of the major advantages of observation as a technique is that it is direct and can contrast with and complement other ways of gathering data. In health and social care, ethnography can be used as a way of accessing and explicating beliefs and practices within an organisation, including those of service users.

Challenges of ethnography

There are undoubted challenges associated with using an ethnographic approach, including the knowledge and skills required of researchers, ethical issues and practical considerations. Robson (2011) noted that ethnography is not a particularly easy research option and to produce meaningful ethnography an understanding of the concepts involved in sociocultural systems is needed.

The ethical implications of using an ethnographic approach have to be acknowledged at the planning stage and, as Hammersley and Atkinson (2007) stated, include informed consent, privacy, harm avoidance and potential exploitation. In health and social care, there is the need to consider the relationship between those watching and those being watched and thought given to the notion of intervention if necessary – for example, if unsafe practice is encountered.

At a practical level, the time involved in collecting the data can be extensive (Robson 2011) and gaining access to an appropriate social setting can be challenging (Bryman, 2012; Hammersley and Atkinson, 2007). There are also concerns about researchers becoming overly involved with their subject groups and 'going native' or contaminating the natural setting and skewing the research. Robson (2011) states that one logical problem is it can be difficult to know what the group's behaviour would have been like *without* the observation taking place, highlighting again the importance of assessing the effects of the researchers' presence (Bryman, 2012; Robson, 2011).

Establishing the credibility of the research and its findings can also be seen as challenging. Fetterman (1998) stated that, as people act on their individual perceptions and those actions have real consequences, the subjective reality of each individual is no less real than a reality that has been objectively measured. Thus, when reporting on and reading ethnographic research, the following questions should be taken into consideration.

- How consistent are the claims with the empirical data?
- How credible is the account to the participants and readers?
- To what extent are the findings relevant to those in similar settings?
- Have the notions of reactivity and reflexivity been acknowledged?
- Does an audit trail exist?

CASE STUDY – JENNI TEMPLEMAN

Critical care nurses experience dying and death in their everyday practice within the fraught and fragile nature of the withdrawal of life-sustaining treatment in intensive care units (ICUs). Improving the quality of end-of-life care within ICUs is of paramount interest to current practice where mortality is high and intensive care personnel, patients and families make the transition from attempting to cure disease and prolong life to providing comfort and allowing there to be dignity in dying and death.

I am undertaking a doctoral research study that explores critical care nurses' experiences following the decision to withdraw life-sustaining treatment in adult patients and how they make sense of the trajectory of dying and death within the culture of this clinical milieu. Ethnography was adopted as a methodology and the written account of the ethnographic narrative incorporated a dramaturgical approach (Goffman, 1959) and Ricoeur's (1984) analytical framework. Research methods included non-participant observation and semi-structured interviews using vignettes.

The choice of ethnography was guided by the epistemological and ontological stances embedded within the research enquiry and that it is pertinent to understanding the 'real world' of nurse practitioners, generating rich qualitative data that supplements and offers depth to evaluations with regard to policy directives and their impact on the staff.

The study depicts how a group of critical care nurses work and explores their beliefs, language, human and physical behaviour following withdrawal of treatment. As the researcher, I have drawn on the constructs of the participants and also applied my own scientific conceptual framework, the so-called emic and etic perspectives. Reflexivity is embedded within the ethnography as an ongoing conversation and story of experiences, while simultaneously living the moment. The written accounts are cultural artifacts of reality and the product of the intermingling of the researcher and the research participants in a certain time and space. The medium of thick description affords readers a sense of the emotions, thoughts and perceptions that participants experience. It deals with the meanings and interpretations of the critical care nurses within their culture and is explicit in the detailed patterns of cultural and social relationships.

It is anticipated that the ethnographic study may complement the existing body of knowledge pertinent to dying and death following withdrawal of life-sustaining treatment within the intensive care milieu and offer meaningful insights for the clinical practice arena.

CONCLUSION

There is much to commend the use of ethnography in health and social care research. Notwithstanding the challenges of putting ethnography into practice as a research method, the value of the approach is that it can reveal great insights into the habits and perceptions of health and social care workers and users and generate theories and solutions to inform and enhance future practice and policies.

FURTHER READING

Hammersley, M. and Atkinson, P. (2007) *Ethnography: Principles in practice* (3rd edn). Abingdon: Routledge.

key concepts in nursing and healthcare research

REFERENCES

Brewer, J.D. (2000) *Ethnography*. Buckingham: Open University Press.

Bryman, A. (2012) *Social Research Methods* (4th edn). Oxford: Oxford University Press.

Fetterman, D.M. (1998) *Ethnography* (2nd edn). Thousand Oaks, CA: Sage.

Geertz, C. (1973) *The Interpretation of Cultures*. New York: Basic Books.

Goffman, E. (1959) *The Presentation of Self in Everyday Life*. London: Penguin.

Hammersley, M. and Atkinson, P. (2007) *Ethnography: Principles in practice* (3rd edn). Abingdon: Routledge.

O'Leary, Z. (2004) *The Essential Guide to Doing Research*. London: Sage.

Polit, D. and Hungler, B. (1999) *Nursing Research: Principles and methods* (6th edn). Philadelphia, PA: Lippincot.

Ricoeur, P. (1984) *Time and Narrative*. Chicago, IL: Chicago University Press.

Robson, C. (2011) *Real World Research* (3rd edn). Oxford: Wiley-Blackwell.

Wolcott, H.F. (1999) *Ethnography: A way of seeing*. Walnut Creek, CA: AltaMira Press.

16 Ethnomethodology

Tom Mason

DEFINITION

'Ethnomethodology' has its roots in sociology and the work of Harold Garfinkel (1967). It is often referred to as microsociology as the method attempts to study the micro features of everyday life by understanding the way that people (actors) order and make sense of the world around them.

The etymology of the term ethnomethodology comes from breaking it down into its three constituent parts 'ethno' (referring to a specific cultural group), 'method' (the practices that this cultural group employ in its everyday life) and 'ology' (from the Greek *logos*, referring to the systematic analysis and description of these methods).

The 'official' definition of ethnomethodology, as coined by Garfinkel (1967: 11) himself, is 'the investigation of the rational properties of indexical expressions and other practical actions as contingent ongoing accomplishments of organised artful practices of everyday life'. However, a non-expert reader will quickly see that this definition is largely impenetrable and may prefer more accessible offerings, such as the systematic study of the ways in which people use social interaction in everyday situations to make sense of what they say and do and, thus, create their own reality.

Here is a brief list of some of the terms used in ethnomethodology.

- **Ethnomethodological indifference** – the attitude of ethnomethodological researchers to the traditional analysis, methods and practices of sociologists to a given area of study. For example, an ethnomethodologist studying crime would be indifferent to traditional aspects of class, social stratification, deviance, role theory and so on. Ethnomethodologists view 'old' spheres in a 'new' light
- **Indexical expressions/indexicality** – a 'segment' of language or behaviour in a specific context that has meaning or sense for those in that specific cultural group. For example, surfers have their own understanding of how to read and ride waves, interpret weather and relay meaning for other surfers. A 'segment' of this communication may be the phrase 'a high roller wave', which conveys sufficient information for other surfers to judge the conditions
- **Rational accounts** – reasoned sense (not common sense) of a particular state of affairs, which describes or explains a social situation
- **Breaching experiment** – an experiment that fractures or breaks the social ordering of a micro aspect of everyday life to reveal or expose the activities that a group engages in to maintain the shared social ordering. For example, Garfinkel requested his student sociologists who were living with their parents to act as lodgers over the weekend. The parents became tense as the rules for the social ordering of being a son or daughter in the family and being a lodger differ significantly from each other
- **Practical accomplishments** – this refers to the assumption that actors in a social setting see action and explanation as a conjoint activity. They see things as they appear to be and the world is 'taken for granted' by them in relation to meaning. For example, a queue forms and has rules, there are sanctions for transgressors of those rules and it has a form of behaviour of its own – this is taken for granted.

DISCUSSION

Like all research methods, ethnomethodology has developed out of other spheres of knowledge and its epistemological base is as much indebted to philosophy as it is to sociology and linguistics. Yet, despite its complex and sophisticated theoretical underpinnings its loci, or focus, is on everyday social situations that are familiar to us all in our cultural group. This Garfinkel termed the mundane. As it is the everyday, or mundane, aspects of life that ethnomethodologists study, which are common to us all, Garfinkel argued that we need strategies to help us see them in a new light or from a fresh perspective.

Historical development

Garfinkel studied under Talcott Parsons at the Harvard Department of Social Relations and was initially influenced by structural functionalism before rejecting the subordination of the social actor in analytical systems theory. He was also influenced by the phenomenology of Alfred Schutz from the Chicago School, but came to believe that his method did not focus sufficiently on the reasoning processes of the competent actors in the social world. Thus, Garfinkel began to define his area of study as the everyday events where those engaging in them are viewed as highly competent and the procedures engaged in are practical accomplishments.

An example of this is the supermarket checkout experience. This is an everyday event that most of us are familiar with and engage in at some point. Garfinkel argues that the management of this situation is a practical accomplishment, making us the experts in the event. As this is a mundane, common event, we fail to 'see' its intricacies, rules, procedures, conventions and so on. The indexical expressions, the queuing behaviour, the stacking of the goods on the conveyor belt, the interactions with the checkout person, the packing of the items into bags and the relations with others in the situation remain largely unnoticed in the mundaneness of the event. If a researcher was to ask a shopper in such a checkout situation what was going on, his or her interpretative account, according to Garfinkel, would be incomplete, although 'good enough for the purposes at hand'.

Applied ethnomethodology

A significant sub-field of ethnomethodology is 'conversational analysis', in which comprehensive recordings and detailed transcriptions of everyday language are made. These have revealed the universal ordering of certain aspects of sociolinguistics, such as 'openings', 'closures', 'turn-taking' and so on. This is not to say that conversational analysis is solely the preserve of ethnomethodology as it has long been studied in numerous branches and disciplines. It has, however, received serious attention in ethnomethodology, from such researchers as Harvey Sacks (1992).

Everyday 'talk', which, in itself, can be understood in its planned sense as communicating a message, is treated differently in ethnomethodology. Not only is the language considered data but also the context in which it is set and the biographies of the interlocutors are treated as contributing to the analysis. As Sharrock (2003: 255) describes it, it is examining 'the conversation in a step-by-step way, to make specific identifications of just what is being said, what is being done by what is being said, and what is being contributed to the conversation by what is being done/said at any specific point'. Imagine the conversation between two surfers mentioned above who may be communicating about the weather but who also may have biographies of surfing, implicitly enthusing each other and urging that they prepare by doing the practical tasks necessary to go surfing in their conversation with each other.

Ethnomethodology has been applied in numerous areas, such as in organisations (Arminen, 2005), science (Woolgar, 1992), theories of the mind (Coulter, 1987) and general sociological theory (Giddens, 1976). It has also been applied in an array of healthcare settings, such as the patient experience (Feder-Alford, 2006), nursing identity (Harper, 2008) and social exclusion in nursing relationships (Allen, 2004) to name but a few.

Social situations have rules and codes of conduct that members of a particular group follow, which gives them a social order. This social order may be different for differing groups, even within the same situation. For example, within a prison there are groups of prisoners as well as prison guards and they both have differing codes by which they manage the prison situation (Wieder, 1974). Both groups, operating via different codes, have a perception of a social reality that also differs according to the meaning given to the context.

These social realities are sometimes difficult to apprehend when they are part of our mundane everyday life and ethnomethodologists believe that we need assistance in appreciating them if we are going to study such social situations. The strategy that they employ is to 'fracture' the social reality of a particular situation, which they do by carrying out what they call 'breaching experiments'. These experiments involve, for example, following different rules, such as acting like a hotel guest at home rather than a son or daughter, mentioned at the beginning of this chapter, thus revealing the rules and ordering of the codes, bringing them into stark relief in order to examine them and form new interpretations.

CASE STUDY

In the supermarket checkout scenario mentioned above, Garfinkel requested his students to undertake their usual shopping and, then, at the point at which the checkout person told them what the final bill was, the students were told to engage in bartering. As this is not the usual code of conduct for a supermarket checkout situation, it fractures the accepted social reality for such an everyday experience.

The students reported that the longer this went on, the greater was the embarrassment of the checkout person and the other shoppers in the queue behind them, who became disquieted. This 'fracturing' initially produced humour, which was followed by irritation and, finally, an official sanction issued by the supermarket's manager.

The students were taught how to observe the behaviour of others and listen to the conversations as the fracturing occurred, thus bringing new insights into the practical accomplishments of the checkout situation.

CONCLUSION

Given the main issues outlined above, it is apparent ethnomethodology is a research approach that is highly relevant to areas of healthcare practice for a number of reasons. Healthcare interactions and practices may become mundane, in the sense that they come to be engaged in automatically, within defined roles (professional, patient) and are task-orientated. This may lead to a form of 'invisibility' of both the codes of conduct and the issues that are raised for healthcare delivery. That such automatic or ritualistic behaviour occurs is well known in healthcare settings, so areas of ethnomethodological interest may reveal new interpretations of traditional situations, such as the nursing 'handover', certain ward routines, skills and competences and nursing reactions in specialised areas such as accident and emergency, mental health settings and midwifery, among many others. Ethnomethodology can bring a new perspective on these healthcare behaviours and reveal alternative levels of interpretation to the superficial rationales for such human actions.

FURTHER READING

Francis, D. (2004) *An Invitation to Ethnomethodology: Language, society and interaction*. London: Sage.

Have, P.T. (2004) *Understanding Qualitative Research and Ethnomethodology*. London: Sage.

Watson, R. (2009) *Analysing Practical and Professional Texts: Directions in ethnomethodology and conversation analysis*. London: Ashgate.

REFERENCES

Allen, D. (2004) 'Ethnomethodology insights into insider–outsider relationships in nursing ethnographies of healthcare settings', *Nursing Inquiry*, 11 (1): 14–24.

Arminen, I. (2005) *Institutional Interaction: Studies of talk at work: Directions in ethnomethodology and conversation analysis*. London: Ashgate.

Coulter, J. (1987) *The Social Construction of Mind: Studies in ethnomethodology and linguistic philosophy*. Houndmills, Basingstoke: Palgrave Macmillan.

Feder-Alford, E. (2006) 'Only a piece of meat', *Qualitative Inquiry*, 12 (3): 596–620.

Garfinkel, H. (1967) *Studies in Ethnomethodology*. Englewood Cliffs, NJ: Prentice Hall.

Giddens, A. (1976) *New Rules of Sociological Method*. Cambridge: Polity Press.

Harper, P. (2008) 'Ethnomethodological ethnography and its application in nursing', *Journal of Research in Nursing*, 13 (4): 311–23.

Sacks, H. (1992) *Lectures on Conversation*. Oxford: Blackwell.

Sharrock, W. (2003) 'Fundamentals of ethnomethodology' in G. Ritzer and B. Smart (eds), *Handbook of Social Theory*. London: Sage. pp. 249–59.

Wieder, D.L. (1974) *Language and Social Reality: The case of telling the convict code*. The Hague: Mouton.

Woolgar, S. (1992) *Science: The very idea*. Abingdon: Routledge.

17 Feminist Research

Elizabeth Mason-Whitehead

DEFINITION

The foundation of contemporary 'feminist research' is in the philosophical standpoint of classical feminist theory. Oakley's (1981: 85) seminal quote sets the scene for the direction of feminist research methodology: 'Ultimately any feminism is about putting women first; it is about judging women's interests (however defined) to be important and to be insufficiently represented in mainstream politics/academia.'

Feminist research builds on this definition and challenges the perceived exploitation and unjust gender inequalities of women, keeping women's interests as the central and first line of enquiry.

- Fundamental to any feminist research study is a theoretical feminist framework from which the area of investigation and the subsequent research method and design are determined
- Understanding feminist epistemology and how it embraces a number of perspectives articulating the perceived unjust treatment of women is an essential requirement prior to engaging with feminist research
- Feminist researchers should identify and justify the feminist position they are adopting in their research. One of the major feminist positions is 'consciousness-raising', which unites women and provides a forum for discussing the specific challenges women face, such as childbirth and abortion. The success of such consciousnessraising can be measured in terms of the political, health and social changes the research prompts
- Researcher and participants are seen as equals in feminist research
- A characteristic of feminist research is that it aims to be participative and the research participants are equal partners and collaborators in it and may have a role in its design, too
- Feminist research is often said to be 'partisan' as it takes the view of improving the social position of women
- A key objective of feminist research is to strive to emancipate the lives of women.
- The subject matter of feminist research is focused on the relationships women have with the rest of society
- Almost exclusively, feminist research uses qualitative methodologies as it is seeking to understand and articulate the lives of women rather than present a quantitative view with statistics

DISCUSSION

The feminist research methodology we practice today has its historical roots in the campaigns to establish equal rights for women in economic, social and political domains. Early political pressure included the 1870 Married Women's Property Act, which allowed women to keep their property once they had married; previously when women married, their property transferred to their husbands. The progress made by the 'women's movement' can be seen in the gradual development from such early campaigns to the development of greater equality, as well as feminist theory, epistemology and research.

Feminist methodology has developed, and continues to develop, from feminist thought and qualitative research methods and changes depending on the times and societies we live in. For example, early feminist research on domestic service (Palmer, 1989) is, thankfully, not relevant to how most of us live now, but there are other more topical studies, such as those on infertility (Caroll, 2012). Ultimately, however, the underlying principles of feminist research remain a constant – the focus is on the experiences of women within a wider social context.

As researchers, we often preoccupy ourselves with 'how to do' research and focus on the practicalities of a particular method and this is especially true of

key concepts in nursing and healthcare research

feminist methodology. We may, for example, embark on a study that is concerned with sexual harassment in the workplace and choose a feminist methodology to do this, with the aim of giving a 'voice' to vulnerable women. While this decision may be entirely appropriate, it is important to understand that feminist methodology is not rooted in 'the how to do' or having the 'tools' to carry out research, but, rather, in our sensitivities regarding the notion of gender, as articulated by feminist methodologists such as Letherby (2011).

Assessing feminist methodology and its contribution to women's experiences raises some positive areas for discussion, but there are also some concerns that such a standpoint presents. On the positive side, the finding and hearing of the 'invisible woman' is a notable achievement of feminist methodology. The position of researchers as equals and people who actively want to tell the stories of their interviewees and may also be involved as participants in the research process, has produced significant studies worldwide that have enabled the 'invisible woman' to become 'visible', such as Fine (1992).

On the negative side, however, criticisms of feminist research include the view that the findings of a feminist study may have been influenced by the researchers' political and social agenda (Thomas and Taylor, 2002).

Figure 17.1 demonstrates the breadth of relationships required of feminist researchers, so each stage of engagement in the research process is considered within a feminist framework.

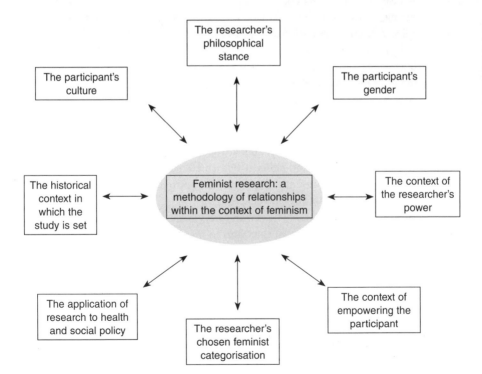

Figure 17.1 Feminist research within a context of significant relationships

Katia has successfully completed her physiotherapy degree and is enjoying her first professional appointment as a physiotherapist, rotating her work in the departments in a large UK teaching hospital. Katia has been asked by the principal investigator of a proposed research study if she would like to join a steering group and offer a physiotherapist's perspective on the reasons for people with chronic orthopaedic conditions missing their hospital appointments.

While Katia is pleased to have been asked to join the group, she is also nervous, as many of the people in attendance will be senior colleagues. Katia meets Indira, professor of clinical research and the principal investigator. Indira detects Katia's anxiety, but puts her at ease, explaining how important her contribution will be and that her relative inexperience will be an advantage, as she will offer fresh ideas.

Katia enjoys the meeting and finds the intellectual discussions stimulating. Katia notes that she is interested in the non-attendance of women for their hospital appointments. Katia has observed that carers are often women who have chronic ill health themselves, often chronic orthopaedic conditions that may be associated with the arduous physical work required to care for those with progressive orthopaedic conditions.

Katia has had a number of conversations with carers as they often ask if she has any advice for their 'bad hip' or 'aching back'. When she has asked why they have not been referred for treatment, they explain that, while they might have had an initial referral from the general practitioner, they have failed to keep their appointments because of their caring commitments.

The steering group has been particularly impressed by Katia's contribution and will take her ideas forward. Katia is introduced to Felicity and Ben, the social scientists of the research team and they ask Katia if she would be interested in developing her idea, with a view to writing a proposal that will be incorporated into the main study.

Over the next few weeks, Katia meets regularly with Felicity and Ben and learns how to write a research proposal that transforms her ideas into a practical investigation. Feminist methodology is the chosen theoretical framework as the researchers want to ensure that the women are not only the main focus of the study but also want to give them a 'voice' by undertaking qualitative interviews.

The research is successful and Felicity, Ben and Katia have had their work published. After a conference presentation, they were approached to submit a research bid for a larger study, expanding on their findings.

The voice of the women carers has clearly now been heard and made accessible to the health and social care community and to carers themselves. Ultimately, this is what feminist research is about, providing evidence to change and reform policy to improve the lives of inequality that many women continue to lead. In this instance, it began with Katia's idea and her determination to overcome her initial anxieties and lack of research experience.

CONCLUSION

Feminist methodology can be most appreciated when it is the catalyst for oppression in women's lives being lifted. While it is now an established research perspective within the qualitative paradigm, it continues to attract criticism for being biased,

key concepts in nursing and healthcare research

lacking in rigour and validity and being out of touch with a world where women are no longer oppressed but enjoy equal rights and opportunities with men. Equally, feminist methodology is praised for exposing and working to overcome the continued inequalities and forms of abuse and exploitation experienced by women, from all backgrounds and all parts of the world.

There seems little likelihood that these opposing views of feminist methodology will ever find common ground, except perhaps in the fact that feminist researchers have provided a coherent voice for previously unheard women in society.

FURTHER READING

Frisby, W., Maguire, P. and Reid, C. (2009) 'The "F" word has everything to do with it: How feminist theories inform action research', *Action Research*, 7 (1): 13–29.

Stanley, E. (ed.) (2013) *Feminist Praxis: Research theory and epistemology in feminist sociology.* Abingdon: Routledge.

REFERENCES

Caroll, K. (2012) 'Infertile?: The emotional labour of sensitive and feminist research methodologies', *Qualitative Research*, 22 August, doi:10.1177/1468794112455039.

Fine, M. (1992) 'Passions, politics and power: Feminist research possibilities', in M. Fine (ed.), *Disruptive Voices*. Ann Arbor, MI: University of Michigan Press. pp. 1– 25.

Letherby, G. (2011) 'Feminist methodology', in M. Williams and W.P. Vogt (eds), *The Sage Handbook of Innovation in Social Research Methods*. London: Sage. pp. 62–9.

Oakley, A. (1981) 'Interviewing women – a contradiction in terms?', in H. Roberts (ed.), *Doing Feminist Research*. London: Routledge. pp 30–62.

Palmer, P. (1989) *Domesticity and Dirt: Housewives and domestic servants in the U.S. 1920–1945.* Philadelphia, PA: Temple University Press.

Thomas, L.R. and Taylor, B.C. (2002) *Qualitative Communication Research Methods.* London: Sage.

18 Grounded Theory

Maureen Deacon

DEFINITION

Lakeman (2011: 928) notes, 'An assumption of grounded theory is that human behaviour is characterised by latent patterns or processes that grounded theory seeks to make visible and explain.' It is these patterns and processes that the researchers work to discover.

'Grounded theory' (GT) is carried out by systematically using flexible methods of data collection and data analysis (Glaser and Strauss, 1967). Charmaz and Mitchell (2001) describe this thus:

- data collection and the analysis of data are performed concurrently (known as 'constant comparative analysis')
- from the beginning of a study, researchers analyse the data for evolving themes and try to understand the fundamental social processes involved
- emergent themes are built into categories that explain how they are integrated within the social processes observed
- a theoretical model is developed that 'specifies causes, conditions and consequences' (Charmaz and Mitchell, 2001: 160).

KEY POINTS

- GT is an approach to research that seeks to develop theory inductively from data
- Data are collected from naturally occurring social settings. These data can be quantitative or qualitative, but tend to be the latter
- GT is used to study social phenomena where no previous theory exists

DISCUSSION

GT and healthcare appear to be natural bedfellows. GT promises a research-based understanding of the real-life work of healthcare practitioners from which theory can be developed and tested. It is this practical orientation to research that makes it so attractive to nurses.

GT is a good example of how research strategies develop as its underpinning philosophy and methods have been argued about for several decades. Indeed, different iterations of GT have been extensively discussed (Parahoo, 2009). These complexities may not be of immediate interest to novice researchers, but such issues need to be considered when learning about the concepts of GT. Take it as a 'health warning' that, while using GT may be a very sensible research strategy, its rigorous application will require careful thought and defence.

Grounded theory unpacked

Understanding the different opinions of influential theorists will enable researchers to defend their approach. These different positions, often referred to as those belonging to first- or second-generation grounded theorists (Morse et al., 2009), influence the research methods employed.

Glaser and Strauss (1967) 'invented' GT and their initial focus was on its methods. Their followers were critical of their lack of attention to the underlying philosophy of knowledge within GT. It is argued that Glaser and Strauss in 1967 were working within a post-positivist philosophy – that is, they assumed that there was a definitive reality to be discovered by an impartial researcher (Birks and Mills, 2011). Their aim was to develop a formal, testable theory.

Second-generation theorists have made their research philosophy more explicit. For example, Charmaz (1995) argued the case for a 'constructivist GT', which places emphasis on the researchers' intersubjective place within the methods employed. In constructivist GT, the theory generated is named 'substantive', meaning that it relates to a specific social setting.

The differences between GT researchers are illuminated via the following case examples, based on a fictitious research aim, which is to identify potentially effective interventions aimed at improving the physical health of people with severe mental illness.

Case example 1

A 'post-positivist GT' approach to this study would make the following assumptions:

- it is possible to improve the physical health of people who are mentally ill
- we should explore practice-based interventions attempting to improve the physical health of people who are mentally ill
- we should examine the ways in which these interventions are being evaluated and the outcomes of those evaluations
- we should engage in a careful literature review, but when we should do so is a matter of debate (it has been argued that doing it prior to data collection and analysis creates bias in terms of what researchers specifically explore, while an alternative view is researchers must understand where their study fits within the wider scholarly field *before* commencing the data collection process)
- we can bring the findings together and, if appropriate, make recommendations for experimental testing of different types of interventions based on the theory generated
- following this, we can state with a degree of certainty that intervention X is more effective than intervention Y (thus producing a formal, generalisable theory).

A 'constructivist GT' approach would share many of these assumptions, but would be more critical. It would regard the 'messiness' of the social world as a matter to be engaged with, rather than screened out as 'variables'. It would consider the intersubjective nature of the data collected. For example, how do the researchers' ideas about what being healthy means affect the kinds of questions they ask? They would question the whole notion of 'effectiveness' and how this is judged.

Despite these different approaches to GT, however, there is good agreement about the basic principles concerning its methods. Let us now return to the case example and apply the constructivist GT approach.

Case example 2

- In the initial phase of our study we interview 12 service users who are understood to have experienced a range of health promotion interventions. The interview guide concerns questions about their experiences and views on what (if anything) has been effective and why they think this was so.

- Following transcription, the early interviews are analysed simultaneously with the continuing interviews. Emergent themes are observed. For example, we note that all the participants interviewed so far are keen and motivated to improve their physical health. We can now observe for this phenomenon appearing in subsequent interviews.
- This early finding (called 'initial' or 'open' coding – the alternative labels reflect the work of different theorists; Birks and Mills, 2011) is consistent across the remaining interviews, with the exception of two. In these 'deviant' cases it is observed that the service users appeared to be acutely mentally unwell. Participant 'Sue' seemed very depressed and stated that she would really rather die than think about her physical health. Participant 'Adam' was difficult to interview. He was unable to engage with the interview topics, preferring to talk repetitively about a conspiracy by MI5 against him. This led the researchers to hypothesise that service users have to be mentally well enough to potentially benefit from any type of general health promotion intervention. A subsequent series of interviews confirm this observation further (known as 'intermediate', 'selective', 'focused' or 'axial' coding).
- These codes are built into categories and sub-categories. So the category 'Being in a position to benefit' has sub-categories of 'Being well enough to benefit', 'Being in a stable enough social position to benefit' and 'Having the resources to benefit'.
- Alongside other categories derived from the interviews and other methods of data collection, the researchers then engage in building a theoretical framework. It is here that they attempt to produce substantive grounded theory (note that the term GT is referring here to a research outcome, whereas previously the term was used to describe a set of research methods). For example, our theory is that an effective health promotion intervention requires the following conditions: a service user who is in a position to benefit from the intervention, an intervention that is acceptable to the service user and an intervention that is applied with the individual's circumstances taken into account.
- This theory could then be further tested, with the aim of producing formal theory.

Grounded theory in healthcare

Parahoo (2009) claims that no qualitative research method has generated more debate than GT. Despite this, Parahoo (2009) argues that many nursing studies claiming to use a GT approach do not distinctively stand apart from other types of qualitative studies. This is because they do not explain the GT methods that they have put into practice or go on to produce formal theory.

Studies using GT often delve into particularly sensitive or controversial aspects of health care. Mangnall and Yurkovich (2010) used GT to explore the use of deliberate self-harm by women held in a US jail. Their analysis led them to develop a model of a circular process of women engaging in deliberate self-harm as a form of emotional pain relief. Deliberate self-harm incidents were regarded negatively within the prison and women were then punished by, among other things, being placed in isolation for substantial periods of time. This would cause them extreme distress, which, in turn, would lead to the need to deliberately self-harm in order to gain relief. Mangnall and Yurkovich (2010) use their findings to make recommendations for forensic nursing practice, but do not propose further development of their theory.

McDonnell and Van Hout (2011) used a GT approach to examine heroin users' experiences of attempting detoxification. While a fascinating study, it dispenses with its GT methods in a very short discussion (13 lines in a 24-page paper!). It is a good example of Parahoo's (2009) criticism discussed above. As in the study by Magnall and Yurkovich (2010), the study by McDonnell and Van Hout (2011) concludes with sensible recommendations for development of the service, but, again, does not explicitly set out a theory that could be subjected to further testing. Note, then, that these researchers have not taken the GT approach to its final point of action.

GT studies also concern more prosaic healthcare matters, but the same intention to 'drill down' into detailed understanding of aspects of healthcare is evident. For example, Livingstone et al. (2011) used GT to explore the experience of amputation in people with diabetes. They clearly illuminate the data analysis process in a table by showing the relationships between data, initial coding, selective coding, categories and a substantive theory of the basic social process. In common with studies using different types of qualitative methods, GT researchers (including Livingstone et al., 2011) often justify their studies by arguing that there is little, if any, existing research in their field of enquiry.

CONCLUSION

It has been argued that GT is a very popular qualitative research strategy in healthcare (Parahoo, 2009). Indeed, Glaser and Strauss (1967) were employed in a school of nursing during their initial work in GT (Birks and Mills, 2011). Why this is the case is easy to understand: it is an approach to research that makes sense to practitioners in their desire to understand and improve complex human processes.

Parahoo (2009: 6) challenges nurses to progress beyond the initial development of a GT study, arguing that:

> Developing a grounded theory is only the first step in the process. The second step is to implement it in practice and the third step is to evaluate and test it. Only then do we know the true worth of the theory. ... Only its use will tell us how 'good' a grounded theory is. Grounded theory has taken a prominent position in nursing research, yet we know little about the effect it has had on nursing practice and on the lives of those for whom nurses care.

The hope is that the next generation of GT researchers will rise to this challenge.

FURTHER READING

Birks, M. and Mills, J. (2011) *Grounded Theory: A practical guide.* London: Sage.
Charmaz, K. (1995) *Constructing Grounded Theory: A practical guide through qualitative analysis.* London: Sage.

REFERENCES

Birks, M. and Mills, J. (2011) *Grounded Theory: A practical guide.* London: Sage.
Charmaz, K. (1995) *Constructing Grounded Theory: A practical guide through qualitative analysis.* London: Sage.
Charmaz, K. and Mitchell, R.G. (2001) 'Grounded theory in ethnography', in P. Atkinson, A. Coffey, S. Delamont, J. Lofland and L. Lofland (eds) *Handbook of Ethnography.* London: Sage. pp. 160–74.
Glaser, B.G. and Strauss, A.L. (1967) *The Discovery of Grounded Theory: Strategies for qualitative research.* New York: Aldine.
Lakeman, R. (2011) 'How homeless sector workers deal with the death of service users: A grounded theory study', *Death Studies,* 35: 925–94.
Livingstone, W., van de Mortel, T.F. and Taylor, B. (2011) 'A path of perpetual resilience: Exploring the experience of a diabetes-related amputation through grounded theory', *Contemporary Nurse,* 39 (1): 20–30.
Mangnall, J. and Yurkovich, E. (2010) 'A grounded theory exploration of deliberate self-harm in incarcerated women', *Journal of Forensic Nursing,* 6: 88–95.
McDonnell, A. and Van Hout, M.C. (2011) 'Forging a path of abstinence from heroin: A grounded theory of detoxification seeking', *The Grounded Theory Review,* 10, (1): 17–40.
Morse, J., Stern, P., Corbin, J., Bowers, B., Charmaz, K. and Clarke, A. (2009) *Developing Grounded Theory: The second generation.* Walnut Creek, CA: Left Coast Press.
Parahoo, K. (2009) 'Grounded theory: What's the point?' *Nurse Researcher,* 17, (1): 4–7.

19   Hermeneutics

Dean Garratt

DEFINITION

The etymology of the term 'hermeneutics' derives from the Greek messenger God Hermes, the Greek noun *hermeneia* translating to 'interpretation' and the Greek verb *hermeneuein* representing the act of translating or interpreting written or spoken language. In Greek folklore, Hermes served as a divine 'mediator' for messages between the Gods, whose communications were often ambiguous and required a rational method of interpretation to discern 'truth' and quell uncertainty.

KEY POINTS

- Hermeneutics involves the study of understanding and interpretation as a process of thinking and being
- The process of interpretation encapsulates both verbal and non-verbal forms of communication as part of a broad-ranging communicative repertoire
- Hermeneutics comprises a variety of traditions and philosophical assumptions

DISCUSSION

Traditionally, the term 'hermeneutics' has been used interchangeably with 'exegesis', employed in biblical hermeneutics to interpret the Bible. A contemporary approach, however, suggests that it can be more widely appropriated as a way of thinking and theory of understanding and, thus, applied to a variety of social science and healthcare contexts. For example, hermeneutic thinking can be employed as a:

- method to elicit and 'produce' data (Kimball and Garrison, 1996; Vandermause and Fleming, 2011)
- methodology to interpret and understand the world around us, especially in clinical research settings (Ajjawi and Higgs, 2007; Vandermause, 2008)
- means of judging the quality and value of qualitative enquiry and healthcare research (Garratt and Hodkinson, 1998; Schwandt, 1999; Smythe et al., 2008).

In more general terms, hermeneutics is not a unitary school, but, rather, encompasses a range of diverse traditions. These both reflect and comprise a variety of different contingent social and cultural histories, with contrasting philosophical antecedents and underpinning assumptions about the nature of knowledge and truth. In their analysis of hermeneutics, Alvesson and Skoldberg (2009) discuss the difference between 'objectivist hermeneutics', popularised by Dilthey (among others) and the tradition of 'alethic hermeneutics', comprising existential, poetic and 'suspicious' forms.

The former – objectivist hermeneutics – represents a point of departure from the precepts of positivism and natural science, but carries the legacy of a sharp dividing line between the 'knowing subject' and 'object of cognition'. This subject–object dualism appeals to a process in which research should endeavour to preserve objectivity and, hence, distance between researchers and researched.

The new 'cultural science', retaining the epistemological currency and methodology of natural science, was markedly different from alethic hermeneutics, which sought to dissolve the binary between subject and object. Instead, hermeneutics became the study of understanding and self-understanding of an ever-changing lifeworld and so, in contrast to cultural science, alethic hermeneutics set out to reveal something 'hidden' through a process of interpretation. For 'existential hermeneutics', this involves revealing 'an original structure of properties buried at the root of our existence, but ... also forgotten', while for 'poetic hermeneu-tics', the purpose of enquiry is to expose 'underlying pattern[s] of metaphor or narrative' (Alvesson and Skoldberg, 2009: 97). The identified hidden quality in the hermeneutics of suspicion 'is something shameful ... in the form of economic interests, sexuality, or power – and therefore repressed' (Alvesson and Skoldberg, 2009: 97). It is the existential variety of philosophical hermeneutics, however, deriving from Heidegger (1995) and Gadamer (1979), on which the remainder of this chapter draws.

The most significant feature of philosophical hermeneutics is its distinctive ontological character. Following Heidegger (1995), one's being in the world – the very thing that is always already there and serves to define who we are – is the element that is most central to our understanding, the understanding informing our every waking moment and, more crucially perhaps, our position as researcher-thinkers. Ontological hermeneutics thus involves a process of being that is conditioned by one's historical circumstances, the social context from which we derive our values, purposes, interests and disposition to act. Put differently, our prejudices or prejudgements about the world.

This tradition and philosophical approach has been usefully applied to the process of hermeneutic listening, which requires us to place our prejudices at 'risk' by means of dialogue in research. As Kimball and Garrison (1996) suggest, the business of interviewing is to engage deliberatively in a process of conversation in which each person, interviewer and interviewee, 'opens' themselves to the other, with a willingness to learn and subsequently change. Such an approach is different from 'empathic listening', for it involves this element of 'risk'. Thus, an interview qua 'dialogical encounter' encourages a process in which we are persuaded, through social interaction, to examine our prejudgements and further question them in order to know ourselves and others in more productive ways. As Gadamer (1979: 299) suggests, the purpose of questioning (for which we might read 'interviewing') is to 'open up possibilities and keep them open'.

On this theme, Schwandt (1999) usefully draws our attention to the phenom-enology of understanding as it relates to the experience of *doing* qualitative research and, thus, coming to understand the possibilities for making sense of our lifeworld hermeneutically. For Schwandt, understanding is an integral part of experience, a process we live through, of learning rather than reading, involving multiple interactions in relations that presuppose openness, dialogue and careful listening. Indeed, such interactions might usefully represent the constituent parts of what it means to do qualitative enquiry in the field of healthcare research. This suggests a form of enquiry that is not only a means of eliciting data through dia-logue or hermeneutic listening but also an heuristic methodology embracing the 'historical, cultural and linguistic context of our practices and our shared being' (Schwand, 1999: 453).

Thus, with the explicit purpose of examining and further understanding the complexity of qualitative data, hermeneutics can reveal particular meaningful insights into the field of healthcare that might later usefully improve our under-standing of professional, clinical practice.

CASE STUDY

A key question that often arises in the context of methodological enquiry is, 'How is the doctoral student of healthcare research able to apply such philosophical concepts to a process of empirical data collection and analysis?' Drawing on the work of a current doctoral student and author (Pritchard, 2012), this section provides a perspective on how the concepts of hermeneutic listening and existential phenomenology have been appropriated to the context of understanding a crucial, but hitherto neglected aspect of healthcare.

Pritchard's small-scale study explored the relationship between patients' anxiety and surgery in the critical, post-operative period. Specifically, this involved the sensitive and emotional subject of seeking to understand 'patients' feelings with regard to the consequences of undergoing surgery for colon cancer'. As Pritchard notes:

> having to face up to life with a colostomy bag or facing chemo or radiation therapy as part of a possible cure can be overwhelming, particularly in terms of side effects from the treatments, such as nausea, vomiting, hair loss and skin lesions. This uncertainty can lead to numerous feelings both positive and negative, which can affect both the physical and psychological makeup of the patient. We as health professionals can affect this process … a positive relationship between the patient and the healthcare professional can be very supportive and helpful both for the patient and his [or her] family, while a negative relationship between the patient and healthcare professional can be destructive.

The specific focus of the study was prompted by the empirical fact that very little is known about this crucial aspect of care – patients' own feelings in the post-operative period following surgery for cancer. Pritchard, with some 27 years of clinical experience as a nurse, was especially interested in *understanding* patients' experiences of 'living with cancer' and, thus, of their perceptions of self in relation to their evolving relationship with family and/or perceived role within family, as well as such deep existential questions and emerging themes as, 'Will this surgery take away who I am? Will I die? What will happen to my family when I die?'

Full ethical approval was granted by the ethics committee of the particular trust concerned before any research was undertaken. Following this, Pritchard selected a purposive sample of patients (reviewing them together with a team of members of staff for suitability) to interview within a week of discharge from hospital.

The interviews, with 15 patients aged 50–80 years, were designed to be exploratory and open-ended, no longer than 60 minutes in duration and, in all cases, be audio-recorded and later transcribed. The opening question, requiring several drafts and iterations, was, 'Can you please tell me about the period after your surgery, from when you woke up until you were discharged?' As Pritchard explains:

> this very open-ended question allowed the patient sufficient scope to explore their feelings and to not limit them to any particular area. It was my intention to limit myself to only two follow-up questions designed solely to encourage the participants to deepen their response, these two responses were 'How did that make you feel?' and 'Would you please tell me more about that?'

19 hermeneutics

99

Here, the crucial element of the enquiry involved a process of listening intently – a form of listening as experience and reflexive engagement in which Pritchard's prejudices (and extensive clinical experience) were wilfully placed at 'risk' in conversational dialogue. Later, this found narrative expression in the articulation of several emerging themes based on patients' experiences of 'coping' with cancer, namely:

- the physical demands of surgery
- the emotional demands of surgery
- the clinical environment
- feelings of loss of control
- the post-operative recovery period.

In each case, the themes developed as part of a reflexive articulation between the self (Pritchard) and the other (the patient), in which the mediated understandings emerged as a product of the 'fusion of horizons' (Gadamer, 1979), a process in which Pritchard became more sensitised, aware and, crucially, more cognisant of the unfamiliar 'other'. As Kimball and Garrison (1996; 56) suggest, 'we broaden our horizons by looking at the landscapes of other people's lives'. In so doing, health professionals may be better disposed, ultimately, to understand and further attend to the clinical needs of their patients.

CONCLUSION

A hermeneutic approach to thinking and listening provides an important means of understanding the clinical needs of patients in, for example, the post-operative period of life-changing surgery. The value of an existential approach, leading to improved understanding and self-understanding of clinical health issues, lies in a more reflexive engagement between the self and the other in ways that are mutually beneficial for both patients and healthcare professionals.

FURTHER READING

Ajjawi, R. and Higgs, J. (2007) 'Using hermeneutic phenomenology to investigate how experienced practitioners learn to communicate clinical reasoning', *The Qualitative Report*, 12 (4): 612–38.

Smythe, E.A., Ironside, P.M., Sims, S.L., Swenson, M.M. and Spence, D.G. (2008) 'Doing Heideggerian hermeneutic research: A discussion paper', *International Journal of Nursing Studies*, 45: 1389–97.

REFERENCES

Ajjawi, R. and Higgs, J. (2007) 'Using hermeneutic phenomenology to investigate how experienced practitioners learn to communicate clinical reasoning', *The Qualitative Report*, 12 (4): 612–38.

Alvesson, M. and Skoldberg, K. (2009) *Reflexive Methodology: New vistas for qualitative research*. London: Sage.

Gadamer, H.-G. (1979) *Truth and Method* (2nd edn). London: Sheed & Ward.

Garratt, D. and Hodkinson, P. (1998) 'Can there be criteria for selecting research criteria?: A hermeneutical analysis of an inescapable dilemma', *Qualitative Inquiry*, 4 (4): 515–39.

Heidegger, M. (1995) *Being and Time*. Oxford: Blackwell.

Kimball, S. and Garrison, J. (1996) 'Hermeneutic listening: An approach to understanding in multicultural conversations', *Studies in Philosophy and Education*, 15: 51–9.

Pritchard, M. (2012) 'A Research Report on the Application of a Selected Research Methodology to a Small Scale Enquiry within a Practice/Professional Setting'. Unpublished doctoral thesis, University of Chester.

Schwandt, T. (1999) 'On understanding understanding', *Qualitative Inquiry*, 5 (4): 451–64.

Smythe, E.A., Ironside, P.M., Sims, S.L., Swenson, M.M. and Spence, D.G. (2008) 'Doing Heideggerian hermeneutic research: A discussion paper', *International Journal of Nursing Studies*, 45: 1389–97.

Vandermause, R.K. (2008) 'The poiesis of the question in philosophical hermeneutics: Questioning assessment practices for alcohol use disorders', *International Journal of Qualitative Studies on Health and Well-being*, 3: 68–77.

Vandermause, R.K. and Fleming, S.E. (2011) 'Philosophical hermeneutic interviewing', *International Journal of Qualitative Methods*, 10 (4): 367–77.

20 Historical Research

Pat Starkey

DEFINITION

'Historical research' in health and social care is the attempt to discover both how and why particular professions and institutions developed. It includes study of legislative change, developments in professional identity and an exploration of the personal experiences of patients, service users and their families and members of staff.

KEY POINTS

- How and why did particular professions and institutions develop?
- What can we know about the experiences of those who worked in them and those who used their services?
- There are many different ways of discovering the past and researchers need to know how to understand and to use them

DISCUSSION

Why bother to find out about the history of our professions?

Just as knowing the history of our own families is both interesting and can help us to understand more about ourselves, knowing about the history of our professions and those who helped to shape them, can help to give us a better understanding of the way that they are structured today. This knowledge is enhanced if we are able to discover what it was like to experience particular professions or institutions, whether as workers, service users or family members.

How can we discover the institutional history of our professions?

There are several ways to explore our past. The principal ones involve the study of official records and publications and recordings of personal experiences. Official papers, photographs, sometimes films and sound recordings are normally kept in repositories known as archives. Ideally, they are stored in carefully controlled physical conditions, free from damp, dust and vermin, and catalogued by specially trained archivists. Material in most archives may be made available to researchers.

Publications, such as professional journals, are generally found in university libraries or the British Library and allow us to appreciate the professional concerns of our predecessors.

Old textbooks may give us an idea of the main interests of those responsible for training staff and help us to understand the ways in which students were trained.

Newspapers can throw light on more general, public discussions and their editorials and sometimes correspondence columns give us some understanding of those social and political pressures that led to changing legislation.

How can we find out about the more personal experiences of people in the past?

The experiences of staff, as well as those of patients and service users, may sometimes be accessed by examining written records, both formal and informal. Personal papers such as letters and diaries may help us to appreciate how some people experienced the care of social workers or hospital staff. Those created by people who worked in the service may give us some insight into their professional lives. Sometimes material like this has been deposited in local record offices or in specialised archives. Other papers may be in the possession of families.

Oral history, which is the recording of interviews with individuals, is another important way of finding out more about the past. This is generally carried out by recording, and then transcribing, interviews.

How can these resources be found and used?

The Internet is an invaluable tool for researchers, but there is so much material online – not all of it either useful or reliable – that it is sometimes difficult to know where to start. The Archive Hub (at: www.archiveshub.ac.uk) is an excellent resource for locating particular records and a good place to start, but it does not list all possible holdings. The sources listed below may help to further narrow down searches.

The official record

This includes records created by Parliament and local authorities. Cabinet papers and similar records of discussion and debate at the highest level of government can be found in the National Archives at Kew, London (online at: www.nationalarchives. gov.uk). The online catalogue gives details of its holdings and instructions for making arrangements to use them. There is a rule that some of these may not be accessed by researchers until 30 years after the events with which they deal (called, not surprisingly, the Thirty Year Rule). Some records may be inaccessible for even longer than that.

Parliamentary debates

The edited verbatim records of Parliamentary debates – generally known as *Hansard*, after the person who first published the records of such proceedings – are published daily and available online (at: www.parliament.uk/business/publications/hansard). This is an invaluable record and source of information about debates that have focused on particular social or economic events, as well as those contributing to the framing of legislation.

Local authorities

Details, including minutes, of meetings are held at local records offices, the addresses of which can be found online, under the name of the relevant local authority, so Bristol Record Office, for example, is at www.bristol.gov.uk/dserve. They may tell us about debates and decisions of, for example, local education or social services committees – decisions that show how the law has been implemented at local level.

Records of professional bodies and trade unions

These are held in a variety of places and many catalogues are available online. For example, the Royal College of Nursing has an online archive catalogue (at: www.rcn.org.uk). The Modern Records Centre at the University of Warwick holds the records of the Trades Union Congress as well as other unions and professional associations, including, for example, the Association of Psychiatric Workers and the British Association of Social Workers (at: www2.warwick.ac.uk/services/library).

Records of charities and voluntary organisations

These are important sources of information. Although some may be found in local record offices, the formal records of other voluntary organisations are often found in other archives. The University of Liverpool, for instance, holds the records of Barnardo's, Action for Children and Family Service Units (now called Family Action) and the catalogues may be consulted online (at: www.sca.lib.liv.

ac.uk/collections/colldescs/social.html). Some large charities, such as the Children's Society (at: www.hiddenlives.org.uk) or NSPCC (at: www.nspcc.org.uk), store their own records and employ their own archivists.

Limits to archival research

Access to personal records is limited for up to 100 years, so it is unlikely that researchers will be allowed to consult case notes, and some organisations place other limits on access. It is normally possible, however, to consult material such as annual reports, official papers relating to meetings and, if you are lucky, some correspondence.

Other useful sources of evidence

Newspapers are vital sources of information and comment. The British Library's collection at Colindale has an online catalogue of its vast holdings (at: www.bl.uk/reshelp/findhelprestype/catblhold/all/allcat.html). Researchers wishing to use these must obtain a reader's ticket and information about doing this is given on its website. Many national newspapers are also available online and may be accessed via university libraries or, occasionally, local record offices, which may hold collections of local newspapers. If these have not been digitised, however, they will have to be viewed on microfilm or microfiche in the library.

Professional journals are valuable sources of information about the way that services have developed and they often record the debates surrounding innovation. Many can be found in university libraries or consulted via the resources of the British Library (at: www.bl.uk/reshelp/findhelprestype/catblhold/all/allcat.html).

Old textbooks demonstrate those aspects of professions and institutions that were viewed as important. The libraries of universities that have taught the relevant academic disciplines may well still hold copies of old textbooks. The British Library is also an important resource when looking for such material (see online at the above address).

The *Oxford Dictionary of National Biography* can be of great assistance to researchers wanting to find out more about people who have made notable contributions to their professions. This is regularly updated and also accessible via many university and public libraries and online (at: www.oxforddnb.com).

The experiences of staff and service users in the past may help us to understand the ways in which treatment and procedures have developed, the changing social and legal context in which our predecessors worked, as well as give us insights into current provision. By interviewing past service users or their families, we can begin to understand their interpretations of their experiences and, taken alongside other evidence, such discussions may help to illuminate particular developments. Whenever possible, interviews should be recorded and transcribed – a process that requires time and patience.

Sometimes letters or diaries are available for study, but researchers must always be aware that memories are unreliable as, inevitably, they record just one side of any one person's experiences. Although they are subjective and need to be read with care, this sort of evidence can nevertheless add colour to a picture built up by other means.

CASE STUDY

Gillian, a nurse in a large university hospital, was keen to learn more about the care of disabled children by a particular voluntary organisation in the 1940s and 1950s.

The organisation's records were in the care of her local university, so she was able to apply for permission to consult them. Although she was not allowed to see personal papers relating to particular individuals, she was allowed to read other documents, which included the organisation's annual reports, records of its committee meetings and other records kept by the home, which specialised in the care of children with physical disabilities. She also found a file that contained some correspondence between the chair of the organisation and the Ministry of Education and another file of newspaper cuttings. In addition, she was able to consult *Hansard* online to follow the debates that had taken place in Parliament about changing legislation and visit the National Archive at Kew, where she examined the records of the Ministry of Education and the Home Office.

In her local records office, she was able to consult the records of the local children's department, to help her understand the ways in which the law was implemented and the relationship between the voluntary organisation and the local authority. Her research also included reading the online versions of some national newspapers and a visit to the British Library's newspaper collection to consult others.

Two people, who had been cared for in a children's home belonging to the organisation, responded to a request for information she put in a local newspaper and allowed her to record interviews with them. One of them showed Gillian letters that she had written to her mother while she was in the home. A woman who had worked at the children's home also responded to Gillian's request and was pleased to help with the research and talk about her training and experience.

With so much material available to her, Gillian was able to ask a number of questions about the provision made for children with disabilities at a particular time and by a particular organisation. Studying the documentation, she thought very carefully about who created the record, for whom and why. She was aware that many official records give only bare details about decisions that have been made and she might have to consult other material in order to find out more about what actually went on. Other records she examined were written very carefully to achieve a particular aim. For example, the annual reports of the voluntary organisation were written for public consumption and tended to stress the positive aspects of its work in order to encourage supporters to continue to give money. She was also able to ask her respondents what it felt like to be a child in such an institution and interview the woman who had worked there and record her story, but was careful to remember that people's memories, too, are not always accurate and may fade.

CONCLUSION

Researching the past requires considerable skill and it may never be possible to get a completely accurate account of the ways in which things have developed. This is because, as noted, records are kept for a specific purpose and will always be phrased very carefully. Also, people's memories fade or become confused, so even first-hand accounts cannot be relied on alone.

FURTHER READING

Black, J. and MacRaild, D. (2000) *Studying History.* Houndmills, Basingstoke: Palgrave Macmillan.
Bornat, J., Perks, R., Thompson, P. and Walmsley, J. (eds) (2000) *Oral History Health and Welfare.* Abingdon: Routledge.

21   Narrative Research

David Coyle

DEFINITION

Listening to, telling and retelling stories is a natural part of our everyday lives and one that plays an often invisible role in our interactions. From our earliest interactions, stories are cast and recast as metaphor and allegory. In our everyday lives, we share stories in our conversations with friends and colleagues about events happening to us or those we know and, in doing so, we create 'narratives'. Stories bind individuals together, creating a sense of who we are and who others are.

Narrative as a research approach, therefore, is naturalistic, common sense and, above all, human. Murray (1999: 49) succinctly places the relationship between social constructs and methodology thus: 'Life and narrative are closely intertwined. While we live lives we simultaneously live within narratives although we may not be aware of these.' Chase (2003: 80) describes the relationship between people and the events that affect their lives as: 'a major way in which people make sense of experience, construct the self, and create and communicate meaning'.

As a methodology, narrative is widely used across professions, including by historians, philosophers and social scientists, psychology and other health professionals (Polkinghorne, 2007). Brooks (1984) states that we are fiction-making machines, by which he means humans are hardwired to understand and communicate experiences via the medium of stories.

KEY POINTS

- Narratives are human, essential to our understanding of the world and the events within it
- Narrative research straddles a range of qualitative methodological approaches
- Narrative studies use semi or unstructured data collection as the means of gathering the storied lives of others
- Narrative and identity can be cast and recast on retelling and the truth of narrative is dependent on the context in which it is offered
- There is no unifying epistemological theory binding narrative approaches
- A narrative approach may focus on the words used, interpretations made of those words or on the performance or interaction of the discourse
- Analysis often takes a structuralist approach, building on Labov (1967, cited in Riessman, 2008)

DISCUSSION

As health professionals, we may not consider assessments to be gathering stories, but they are just that. Via assessment, we are attempting to uncover the series of events or story that has led the patient or user to the point where he or she is sat in front of us. We are asking for their account or journey from health to illness or from security to distress or from trauma to a form of recovery.

Stories can reveal a rich source of information and insight if we extend the notion of narrative as illuminating people's perceptions of their situations. Narrative research is the process of listening to and making meaning from storied constructions, which becomes both the method and the approach. Narrative as an approach to healthcare research can create powerful and compelling accounts of experiences of health and illness that directly influence care delivery and organisation (Holloway and Freshwater, 2007). In a time when healthcare professionals are being compelled to move towards a more patient-focused delivery of care, the narrative approach now has its time.

Edwards (2006) points out that narratives or stories can offer more than simple chronological accounts. Stories can provide the participants' explanations of experiences, events and the role of themselves and others within those events. A breadth and diversity exists within narrative research that is reflected across the range of professionals employing the methodology. Irrespective of the many professional groups or their approaches to the use of narrative story work, the method has a strong place within healthcare research. It gains further meaning and importance when set against Murray's (2008: 53) assertion that, 'Illness gains meaning through the stories we tell about it. In diagnosis, during its course, and after the illness has ended or at least subsided, we attempt to bring order to the crisis by constructing a story.'

Gathering stories as a method for data collection might be used within a narrative per se or may be utilised by other qualitative schools and subjected to their epistemological analysis. For instance, phenomenologists seek first-person lived experience from third-party perspectives using interpretative re-enactment of the dialogue via transcripts or by placing text within a different context to arrive at analysis (Lai, 2010). Discourse analysts explore the performance of the participants alongside the text or transcripts, noting discrepancy and prosodic differences.

Narrative research's flexibility is one of its strengths, allowing for a multitude of settings, participants and approach. Conversely, such flexibility constitutes methodological weakness for some. Riessman (1993) is clear about placing narrative beyond the positivists' gaze and, instead, permits diversity as a means of understanding others. Caution should always be taken, however, and it should be borne in mind that truth in narrative, as in most forms of research or enquiry, is elusive so we should always recognise:

> Narrative analysts, in practice, approach the issue of truth differently. Some assume that language represents reality: The narrative clauses recapitulate experience in the same order as the original events (Labov and Waletzky (1967), cited in Riessman (1993: 18)). Others, influenced by phenomenology, take the position that narrative constitutes reality. It is in the telling that we make real phenomena in the stream of consciousness. (Riessman, 1993: 22)

Narrative research has to go beyond stories shared in our everyday lives, however. Stories need to be collected and retained. They have to be analysed, with rigour applied in order that they can be valued as part of a meaningful applied research method.

Approaches for analysing narrative data are varied, but whichever one is chosen, the principles of good data collection apply. Most often, an open-ended interview approach is used, with the researcher recording the interview to later be transcribed and analysed. The analysis of stories can be best understood when conforming to an established and recognisable pattern. Traditional narratives have a beginning, middle and end, for example. Indeed, Charon (2006) defines temporality as a component of narratives – the temporal order of things, with events having a beginning, middle and end.

Riessman (1993) cites Labov's (1967) six components of a 'fully formed narrative', presented as a structural analysis of it. Researchers, in seeking to understand the events in the subjects' lives will seek an 'abstract', presented as a summary or focus. A story will have an 'orientation', setting the events in a place and time, including who was involved and their places in relation to the teller. From this point, a story will involve what Aristotle (cited in Brooks, 1984) described as a *Mythos*, or plot, which forms a sequence of events, and Labov terms a 'complicating action'. Within the complicating action, plots may twist or relate to pivotal moments. Labov then turns to the soul of narratives, which is when tellers step back from the action and reflect on their 'evaluation' of their stories and plots. A story finishes with a 'resolution' – that is, the consequences or results of the plot are stated – and, finally, with a 'coda', which is when a narrative is brought back to the present.

Riessman states that most narrative researchers use Labov's components as either a starting point or point of reference. She is clear also that, while Labov considered the components above to be present in a fully *formed* story, narratives may not be complete and disobey the order set out above. Indeed, when interviewing participants on subjects for which the emotional content is high, narrative may be confused or disjointed in retelling.

Narrative plot – when tellers or characters within stories conform to tragic, heroic, satirical or comedic structures – is a common frame (Frye, 1957, cited in Murray, 2008). The tellers may recount narratives constructing notions of suffering or great struggle (Kelly, 1994, cited in Bury, 2001 and Charmaz, 1999).

CASE STUDY

The narrative method was used in this case to capture accounts of mental health service users with psychosis accessing individual budgets.

The approach utilised open-ended interviews on two occasions, focusing on each person's journey through the mental health service. The interviews lasted between one and half and two hours and were later transcribed. Analysis was influenced by the work of Bury (2001), who explores more than the traditional Labovian structure by attempting to understand the contingent moral and core narratives of a person's story. Bury's approach first seeks a 'contingent narrative' or understanding of an event and the causes or contributory factors leading to the illness. Next, 'moral narratives' may be seen, which describe attributional components of the self in the context of societal factors (here, ideas of self-harming, worthiness and punishment might exist beyond the individual) (Bury, 2001). In this study, many respondents had histories of substance misuse and cast their actions as attributional to their current difficulties. Regarding the 'core narrative', this is a person's understanding of their narrative as conforming to classic or genre scripts (Murray, 2008).

An additional analysis was applied, based on the work of Robinson (1990) – that of using 'regressive narratives'. These relate to when lived experience is perceived as deteriorating. A 'stable narrative' is when a person's experience is static or else a sense of being stuck might be conveyed.

The final filter used in this work explored the possibility of a 'progressive narrative', which is when life is perceived as moving forward. Each interview produced data that was read and reread within Robinson's construct. Table 21.1 shows how the story work reflected a progressive narrative of constructing hope and recovery as the user progressed through the service.

Table 21.1 Service users' experiences of the individual recovery budget (Coyle, 2011)

Hope of recovery	Positive self-direction
A position of dependence	Towards authorship of their future
Having been assessed	Cocreation of person-centred plans

CONCLUSION

Riessman (1993) states that the issues of truth and authenticity in narrative can be contested as a single narrative does not exist. Depending on the epistemological frame of the listener or researcher, different understandings or truths will emerge. For researchers employing a narrative approach, the mantra of being clear and transparent in determining the framework and processes of analysis is key.

Narrative methodologies represent a broad church, allowing stories of experiences to be given a voice, expression and to breathe. There is no single narrative and researchers will be reflexive in their approach, recognising times when their own frame for comprehension and construction may speak over the stories they are seeking to hear and addressing that.

FURTHER READING

Riessman, C.K. (2008) *Narrative Methods for the Human Sciences*. London: Sage.
Murray, M., (2008) 'Narrative psychology', in J. Smith, *Qualitative Psychology: A practical guide to research methods*. London: Sage.

REFERENCES

Brooks, P. (1984) *Reading for the Plot Design and Intention in Narrative*. Cambridge, MA: Harvard University Press.

Bury, M. (2001) 'Illness narratives: Fact or fiction?', *Sociology of Health and Illness*, 23 (3): 263–85.

Charmaz, K. (1999) 'Stories of suffering: Subjective tales and research narratives: Keynote address at the Qualitative Health Research Conference, February 19–21, 1998, in Vancouver, British Columbia', *Qualitative Health Research*, 9 (3): 362–82.

Charon, R. (2006) *Narrative Medicine: Honouring the stories of illness*. Oxford: Oxford University Press.

Chase, S. (2003) 'Learning to listen: Narrative principles in a qualitative research methods course', in R. Josselson, A. Lieblich and D. McAdams (eds), *Up Close and Personal: The teaching and learning of narrative research*. Washington, DC: American Psychological Association. pp. 79–99.

Coyle, D. (2011) 'Impact of person-centred thinking and personal budgets in mental health services: Reporting a UK pilot', *Journal of Psychiatric and Mental Health Nursing*, 18 (9): 796–803.

Edwards, D. (2006) 'Narrative analysis', in A. Jaworski and J. Coupland (eds), *The Discourse Reader* (2nd edn). Abingdon: Routledge. pp. 227–39.

Holloway, I. and Freshwater, D. (2007) *Narrative Research in Nursing*. Oxford: Blackwell.

Lai, K.A.C. (2010) 'Narrative and narrative enquiry in health and social sciences', *Nurse Researcher*, 17 (3): 72–84.

Murray, M.P. (1999) 'The storied nature of health and illness', in M.P. Murray and K. Chamberlain (eds), *Qualitative Health Psychology: Theories and Methods*. London: Sage. pp. 47–63

Murray, M. (2008) 'Narrative psychology', in J. Smith, *Qualitative Psychology: A practical guide to research methods*. London: Sage. pp. 111–32.

Polkinghorne, D.E. (2007) 'Validity in narrative research: The future of narrative research', *Qualitative Inquiry*, 13 (2): 1–16.

Riessman, C.K. (1993) *Narrative Analysis: Qualitative Research Methods*, Vol. 30. London: Sage.

Riessman, C.K. (2008) *Narrative Methods for the Human Sciences*. London: Sage.

Robinson, I. (1990) 'Personal narratives, social careers and medical courses: Analysing life trajectories in autobiographies of people with multiple sclerosis', *Social Science and Medicine*, 30 (11): 1173–86.

key concepts in nursing and healthcare research

22 Observational Research

Sandra Flynn

DEFINITION

'Observation' is a method that allows researchers to directly observe individuals in their natural settings (Carlson and Morrison, 2009) or in a controlled environment (Langdridge and Hagger-Johnson, 2009). Observation has been defined as (Angrosino, 2007: 98):

> a tool of social inquiry in which activities and relationships of people in the study community are perceived through the five senses of the researcher.

Observational methods require researchers to watch and record human behaviour and related events and objects, interpreting and evaluating the data gathered (Waltz et al., 2009).

Observational studies in nursing and healthcare research play a pivotal role when information is sought on the effectiveness of treatment and care, patient-reported outcomes and costs in real-life locations (Langham et al., 2011).

KEY POINTS

- In observational studies, researchers seek to observe a series of events in a natural setting or in a controlled environmental setting
- The two main types of observation are structured and unstructured
- Participant or non-participant observer roles may be assumed, according to the extent to which an investigator controls the environment
- Measurement using observation is prevalent in qualitative research and can be used in quantitative research
- In observational research, observing what does *not* happen is just as important as observing what *does* happen

DISCUSSION

Observation as a research method has the distinct advantage of being able to directly access the 'lived experience' of the individual. Frequently referred to as 'field research' or 'fieldwork' (Spradley, 1980), the method is often used by anthropologists, sociologists and political scientists. It can provide a rich, detailed description of phenomena that is unconstrained by predetermined concepts and categories. Observation methods can be particularly helpful when describing complex behaviour and formulating hypotheses about them and about relationships between different components or elements (DeWalt and DeWalt, 2010) such as, for example, a patient's perception of staff behaviour.

Observational studies focus on the direct observations of researchers, who, in turn, aim to immerse themselves in the world of the subjects being studied, with the intention of seeing the world as the subjects see it, rather than as the researchers perceive it to be. The researchers record the observed events, conversations and behaviours by compiling field notes – their primary method of capturing data from observation (DeWalt and DeWalt, 2010). The aim of observational research is to produce knowledge (empirical and theoretical) about distinct issues that can then be used by others in a number of ways – for example, the measurement of the use of resources in hospitals.

In healthcare, observation is considered the most important data-collection method, particularly in studies focusing on human behaviour, and can be used as a stand alone method or in conjunction with others (Parahoo, 2006).

Observational studies are considered non-interventional. In healthcare, this means that the care and treatment of patients is performed naturally in practice without influence from the researchers or the study. Observational settings reflect naturalistic as opposed to artificial circumstances. As such, individual lives, conversations and behaviours are not regulated by particular rules or regulations, allowing for improved observation of the natural progression of disease processes (Bang, 2010). This is important as the ability to observe natural events and occurrences enables healthcare professionals to evaluate the effectiveness of care and treatment in patient populations.

Structured observation

'Structured observation' is said to be predetermined, in that researchers decide in advance which aspects of phenomena to observe. It is a way of looking for something and is useful in helping researchers to ascertain whether or not the aspects of phenomena are present and to what extent (Gillham, 2008).

Structured observation requires the use of a checklist or schedule to record observations. Most researchers will devise categories that are allocated codes to help with the recording and analysis of the data collected. Structured observation can be similar to a survey, where certain types of behaviours, activities or interactions are looked for.

This type of observation is usually performed by researchers who are operating from a 'positivist' perspective – that is, they believe it is possible to clearly define and quantify behaviours. Quantitative research often employs the use of structured observation.

Unstructured observation

'Unstructured observation' simply involves researchers recording what they see or hear. It is a way of looking at a situation to observe something that is naturally occurring. Researchers approach unstructured observation with no predetermined ideas. The process begins with the selection of a setting and obtaining access to it, observations are made, then recorded. As such studies evolve, so the nature of the observation changes, becoming sharper and more focused. This, in turn, leads to the formulation of purer research questions and selected observations until theoretical saturation is reached (Adler and Adler, 1994). Observation conducted as part of qualitative research is often unstructured.

In unstructured observation, researchers are usually acting from a 'critical' perspective, as the focus is on understanding the meaning the studies' participants attribute to behaviour or events within the contexts observed (Gillham, 2008).

Observation participation

The environmental opportunities for observers are many. Gold (1958) discusses the variations that exist in the roles undertaken by the researchers, ranging from complete observer, the participant as observer, the observer as participant to complete participant. The roles that the researchers choose to adopt are subject to change throughout the fieldwork and can be influenced by the study setting and the research (Hammersley and Atkinson, 2007).

Participant observation is a way of performing ethnographic research, placing researchers in the heart of, and interacting with, the community under study (Angrosino, 2007) – in other words, it is a process that allows researchers to learn about the behaviour and activities of the people being studied in their natural surroundings. In so doing, it enables researchers to gain a deep understanding of a community's intricacies and inner workings that cannot be obtained from the literature (DeWalt and DeWalt, 2010).

Participant observation allows researchers to completely submerge themselves in an environment in order to understand and 'become' members of the culture without inflicting their own social reality on that culture (Layder, 1992). The researchers live within a certain context, maintain relationships with people, participate in activities, while taking extensive and intricate notes on the experience. The process involves more than pure observation, incorporating interviews and analysis of documents so that knowledge is acquired of the social phenomena from the perspective of the subjects. Gold (1958: 217) provides a description of the four observer categories, given in Table 22.1.

Observation can be used as part of a mixed methods approach, whereby other approaches are used to also gather information. Observational methods can form part of an exploratory method for quantitative research or used in triangulation, providing validation for other qualitative research.

CASE STUDY

Michelle is currently undertaking a research study as part of her degree. She has submitted a research proposal and obtained ethical approval for the study, which involves observing the interactions between clinical and clerical staff in an outpatient department at her local district general hospital. Her method involves

Table 22.1 Categories of observation (Gold, 1958: 217)

Role	Advantages	Disadvantages
Complete participant The true identity and purpose of researcher is kept hidden	• Does not influence natural events being studied • Data validity is increased (Bernard, 2011) • Reduces problems associated with observer effects	• May become involved in dangerous practices or behaviours • A level of deceit • Risk of overidentification with the studies' participants, known as 'going native' (Frankenberg, 1982) • Infringes the principle of 'informed consent' (Burgess, 1989)
Participant as observer Researcher gains access to research setting, usually having a non-research reason for being part of the research environment	• Observes from standpoint of full group member • More observation than participation • Researcher and participant aware that relationship is founded on research activity	• Time needed to build trust between researcher and participant • Informant may become too much of an observer • Researcher may overidentify with informant
Observer as participant Observing without being a member	• Ability to concentrate on data collection • Improved observation and understanding of events • Researcher's role is strictly research focused • Less risk of researcher 'going native'	• Level of information is controlled • Trust in researcher needed • Risk of misunderstanding of observed events due to short, one-off visits
Complete observer Researcher does not take part in research setting	• Observation is unobtrusive • Unknown to participants	• Lower data validity (LeCompte and Goetz, 1982) • Purpose of observation is not revealed

gathering data on how effective the clinic administration system is and how efficiently this is used by all the members of staff.

Michelle is using observation to collect some of the data for the study. Importantly, all the members of staff have been fully informed of her observational research and been given the option to take part or decline to participate in the study. Michelle has given a small seminar presentation to explain her research rationale and anticipated outcomes.

During the observation periods, Michelle attends the outpatient department waiting area and sits where she feels she is able to observe most of the events. Michelle takes field notes during and after the observed sessions and, once she has written up her findings, she will present a report to the outpatient department manager. Together, they will examine the findings to see where changes can be made to enhance the patient experience. The data collection is thus achieved in line with the aims and ethical considerations of the study.

CONCLUSION

Observational research can provide important information for clinical and research purposes. Observation can be used in qualitative and quantitative research studies and as part of experimental and non-experimental designs. The aims of a research study can influence the degree of researcher participation within the research community and environment.

FURTHER READING

Polgar, S. and Thomas, S.A. (2007) *Introduction to Research in the Health Sciences* (5th edn). Edinburgh: Churchill Livingstone.

Pope, C. and Mays, N. (2006) *Qualitative Research in Health Care* (3rd edn). Oxford: Wiley-Blackwell.

REFERENCES

Adler, P. and Adler, P. (1994) 'Observational techniques', in N.K. Denzin and Y.S Lincoln (eds), *Handbook of Qualitative Research*. Thousand Oaks, CA: Sage. pp. 377–92.

Angrosino, M. (2007) *Doing Ethnographic and Observational Research*. London: Sage.

Bang, H. (2010) 'Introduction to observational studies', in D.E. Faries, A.C. Leon, J.M. Haro and R.L. Obenchan (eds), *Analysis of Observational Health Care Data Using SAS*. Cary, NC: SAS Institute Inc. pp. 3–19.

Bernard, H.R. (2011). *Research Methods in Anthropology* (5th edn). Lanham, MD: Alta Mira Press.

Burgess, R.G. (ed.) (1989) *The Ethics of Educational Research*. London: Falmer Press.

Carlson, M.D.A. and Morrison, S.R. (2009) 'Study design, precision, and validity in observational studies', *Journal of Palliative Medicine*, 12 (1): 77–82.

DeWalt, K.M. and DeWalt, B.R. (2010) *Participant Observation: A guide for fieldworkers*. Lanham, MD: AltaMira Press.

Frankenberg, R. (1982) 'Participant observers', in R.G. Burgess (ed.), *Field Research: A sourcebook and field manual*. London: Allen & Unwin. pp. 50–52.

Gillham, B. (2008) *Observation Techniques: Structured and unstructured approaches (real world research)*. London: Continuum.

Gold, R. (1958) 'Roles in sociology field investigation', *Social Forces*, 36: 217–23.

Hammersley, M. and Atkinson, P. (2007) *Ethnography: Principles in practice* (3rd edn). Abingdon: Routledge.

Langdridge, D. and Hagger-Johnson, G. (2009) *Introduction to Research Methods and Data Analysis in Psychology*. Harlow: Pearson Prentice Hall.

Langham, S., Langham, J., Goertz, H. and Ratcliffe, M. (2011) 'Large-scale, prospective, observational studies in patients with psoriasis and psoriatic arthritis: A systematic and critical review', *BMC Medical Research Methodology*, 11, 32.

Layder, D. (1993) *New Strategies in Social Research*. Cambridge: Polity Press.

LeCompte, M.D. and Goetz, J.P. (1982) 'Problems of reliability and validity in ethnographic research', *Review of Educational Research* 52 (1): 31–60.

Parahoo, K. (2006) *Nursing Research: Principles, process and issues* (2nd edn). Houndmills, Basingstoke: Palgrave Macmillan.

Spradley, J.P. (1980) *Participant Observation*. New York: Holt, Rinehart & Winston.

Waltz, C.F., Strickland, O.L. and Lenz, E.R. (2009) *Measurement in Nursing and Health Research* (4th edn). New York: Springer.

23 Phenomenology

David Coyle

DEFINITION

'Phenomenology' – from the Greek, meaning 'that which appears' – is mostly interpreted as exploring the lived experience of another as experienced by that person. Phenomenology as a means of understanding the experiences of others can produce high-quality data and insights that assist healthcare workers in responding well to those they serve. In qualitative studies, phenomenology is often involved as many studies attempt to obtain a first-person perspective from a third-person vantage point.

Widely used across domains, including psychology, medicine, physiotherapy, occupational therapy and nursing, phenomenology represents an honest attempt to understand and use the worldviews and interpretations of others to better respond to user needs and improve delivery approaches. The method is naturalistic, in so far as it sits within classic traditions of constructivist and postmodern ideas of identifying and defining what it means to be and what experiences are shared.

KEY POINTS

- Phenomenology is used by many researchers in nursing and allied healthcare as a means of exploring and articulating the experiences of others, illuminating the impacts of disease, health and resilience
- 'Husserlian phenomenology' is the original iteration of an approach that seeks the meaning of experiences and to identify the essence of those experiences. The approach takes an epistemological stand in endeavouring to view with an objective lens the world of others unencumbered by preconceptions and bias
- 'Heideggerian phenomenology' or 'hermeneutic phenomenology', based on an ontological standpoint, engages researchers as part of the enquiry, requiring that the investigators recognise their effect and engagement with the research subject and process
- 'Interpretative phenomenological analysis' (IPA) is a contemporary approach that is similar to hermeneutic and Husserlian methods, but employs clear processes for framing and analysis

DISCUSSION

The use of phenomenology in healthcare research has become almost ubiquitous. Phenomenology is cited as the research method in countless articles, though it is suggested that in terming some of them 'phenomenological studies', the researchers are misusing the term and misidentifying the studies as such.

'Method' and 'approach' in phenomenology are used interchangeably, with little thought as to their origin, meaning and, therefore, usefulness. Many texts and approaches exist relating to the use of phenomenology (such as: Colaizzi, 1978; Giorgi, 1985; Van Kaam, 1969), with Streubert and Carpenter (2010) providing a clear and helpful overview.

Philosophical subtlety and methodological standpoints can make phenomenological comprehension especially challenging for novice researchers, but, combined with language that is often difficult, the task facing all researchers embarking on phenomenological work can be daunting. Here, therefore, we will seek to, first, provide an overview of the two pillars of phenomenology – Husserl and Heidegger, whose work underpins most of what has followed – and then discuss a contemporary iteration of phenomenology – interpretative phenomenological analysis – that, in part, bridges transcendental and existential–hermeneutic phenomenology.

Transcendental phenomenology

Edmund Husserl (1859–1938) is largely seen as the founder of the phenomenological philosophy and approach. Trained as a scientist and mathematician, Husserl was influenced by the philosophical writings of René Descartes and Cartesian dualism – that is, the mind–body split. The essence of this idea is that the mind is separated from the 'container' of the body. Husserl's aim was to explore the essence of what experience is, as opposed to what the experience represents. This separation between the world of objects and sensation is what Coch (1995: 828) describes as:

> the study of phenomena as they appear through the consciousness. Central to Husserl's approach was the fundamental recognition of experience as the ultimate ground and meaning of knowledge.

Through rigorous analysis and reanalysis, the aim of transcendental phenomenology is to arrive at the essence of something or of an experience (Crotty, 1996). Researchers have to engage in a process of filtering cultural, personal presumptions to arrive at the essence of the experience itself, so the being of something can be separated from the conceptualisation of that thing.

This transcendental approach to reality was envisaged as the first science and an attempt at finding truths. Thus, the paradigm seeks objectivity at its origin and parallels, to a degree, scientific reductionism, though Husserl rejected experimental science in favour of the philosophical and existential paradigm.

Important within transcendental or descriptive phenomenology is the process by which the known sense or common sense is recognised and managed. To Husserl it was necessary to avoid *what* it is that is being observed becoming obscured by what is already known. The common sense of daily life, the unattended to and almost automatic actions individuals engage in as they go about their daily lives obscure the essence of experience that was sought by Husserl.

The process known as 'eidetic reduction', in which only the essential constituents of the observed phenomena would be described, therefore forms the aim of this first phenomenology. An example of eidetic reduction is candle wax as it may take on differing shapes, textures and forms, be melted or solid, but it is still, chemically and structurally, wax.

The point for phenomenologists in the Husserlian tradition is the notion that many human experiences are universal and, as such, can be observed and described in a context free from culture, history or situation. This eidetic form creates the scientific gaze Husserl sought for phenomenology – that human experience and its universality transcends the individual, creating an essence for description and study.

For an enquirer to observe and attend to the essence or first principle of the subject, 'intentionality' or focus are essential. Focusing on the topic, the mundane and everyday are thrown into sharp relief. Crucially, in transcendental phenomenology, a process of casting aside, temporarily, what is common sense or preknowledge is required. Husserl termed the process *'epoché'* or bracketing. It involves enquirers acknowledging their pre-existing understanding and consciously setting this knowledge or bias aside, revealing the remaining essence of the experience. Some undertaking descriptive phenomenology would advocate that, as part of this bracketing process, researchers should avoid undertaking a detailed literature review so as to arrive at the material fresh (Lopez and Willis, 2004).

Hermeneutic phenomenology

Martin Heidegger (1889–1986) was a student of Husserl's, but his philosophical work led him to diverge from Husserl and develop a separate strand of phenomenology. The result – 'hermeneutic' or 'interpretative phenomenology', also known as 'existential phenomenology' (Coch, 1995).

For Heidegger, researchers need to be within the world that is being investigated – this is an intrinsic and necessary part of investigation – so he dismisses the construct of bracketing as a separation between the researchers' fore-knowledge and the research subjects' experience as not being possible. The researched and researcher should inhabit the same space, as culture, meaning and essence exist before a person is aware of them and such culture predates any observation.

Thus, phenomenology for Heidegger is essentially a social action and one in which science and understanding of behaviour are coproduced and, therefore, any attempt at *epoché* would be pointless. As beings-in-the-world (Walters, 1995), we are inescapably a part of the lived world. As humans, we are in what Heidegger termed *'Dasein'* – an ordinary German word meaning 'being there' (Holloway and Wheeler, 2010), a state of asking *who* we are rather than *what* we are.

Central to the approach is hermeneutics, which, when applied to research work, results in an interpretation of what culture or historicity or fore-perception existed in the world before our awareness of it. This assertion may seem difficult, but it does represent one of the fundamental differences between Husserl and Heidegger. As seen above, for Husserl, objective distancing from phenomena can be achieved via *epoché*, the suspension of bias and knowledge. For Heidegger, such separation is not possible as we are inextricably connected to being-in-the-world and can only interpret what already exists.

Coch (1995) describes eloquently the phenomenon of 'constitutionality' and the 'hermeneutic circle', both of which are central to the philosophy and practice of Heidegger's phenomenology. Through engagement with the hermeneutic circle, sense and meaning are constituted and meaning found.

Interpretative phenomenological analysis (IPA)

'Interpretative phenomenological analysis' (IPA) (Smith et al., 2009) is primarily concerned with the question of understanding others' experiences and the sense they make of it. Originating in a psychology tradition, it is a relatively recent development. The work uses ideas from the phenomenology tradition (Williams et al., 2010) and, in many aspects, is closely related to the hermeneutic tradition, concerning itself with the emic of personal meaning and interpretation for the individual.

The method involves researchers in interpreting both phenomena and discovering similarities by generating themes. The etic of wider observation, which is close to Husserlian phenomenology, and the objective of eidetic reduction, seeing the experience as a separate object, are both used within IPA. Trying to balance the differing standpoints of traditional phenomenology, IPA manages to provide a balanced position between disparate traditions.

IPA, in addition, promotes an idiographic stance, seeking to fully understand the unit of experience for the subject before understanding the experiences of others within the sample. This process prevents a rapid and potentially premature summation of the etic being studied. To this end, the role played by researchers is central within the process of IPA in that their understanding of the experiences observed while undertaking data collection and during analysis are given voice and contribute to the formation of description and meaning.

The IPA approach is gaining popularity, reaching beyond its beginnings in psychology to healthcare settings ranging from dementia care, mental health and addiction to palliative care (Reid et al., 2005). Those wishing to explore IPA further may, in the first instance, see the IPA's website (at: www.ipa.bbk.ac.uk).

Below, Coch (1995) provides the essential differences between the method – focused or epistemological approach of Husserl set against the ontological existential world view from Heidegger. IPA has been included to show where this sits alongside and against the traditions of Heidegger and Husserl.

Sample size and data collection in phenomenology

In keeping with most forms of qualitative methodology, sample size in phenomenology is not governed by the demands of ensuring generalisability and applicability to whole populations. The work at hand is concerned with detailed accounts and understanding of phenomena and the meaning of those experiences for those concerned.

Table 23.1 The essential differences between the phenomenological approaches of Husserl, Heidegger and interpretative phenomenological analysis (IPA) (adapted from Coch, 1995: 832)

Husserl	Heidegger	IPA
Transcendental phenomenology	Hermeneutic phenomenology	Takes on both etic and emic (the object and culture)
Epistemological	Existential–ontological	Both, though mostly ontological in its stance
Epistemological questions of knowing	Questions of experiencing and understanding	Both, though leaning towards understanding
How do we know what we know?	What does it mean to be a person?	What it means to be a person and observing
Cartesian dualism, mind–body split	*Dasein* (being there)	Being there
A mechanistic view of the person	Person as self-interpreting being	Person as self-interpreting being
Mind–body person lives in a world of objects	Person exists as a being in and of the world	Person exists as a being in and of the world
Ahistorical	Historical	Both
Unit of analysis is the meaning given by the subject	Unit of analysis is the transaction between the situation and the person	Both and the meaning for researchers
What is shared is the essence of the conscious mind	What is shared is culture, history, practice, language	What is shared is culture, history, practice, language
Starts with a reflection of mental states	We are already in the world in our prereflective selves	Starts with a reflection of mental states
Meaning is unsullied by the interpreters' own normative goals or view of the world	Interpreters participate in making data	Interpreters participate in making data
Participants' meaning can be reconstituted in interpretive work by insisting that data speak for themselves	Within the already known structure of understanding, interpretation can only make explicit what is already understood	Within the already known structure of understanding, interpretation can only make explicit what is already understood
Claim that adequate techniques and procedures guarantee validity of interpretation	Establish own criteria for trustworthiness of research	Audit trail similar to Heidegger's, though more rigorously defined
Bracketing defends the validity of interpretation against self-interest	The hermeneutic circle (background, co-constitution, pre-understanding)	Co-constituting with analysis of discourse outside of phenomenology

Phenomenology, then, whether Husserlian, Heideggerian or IPA, is concerned about the appropriate people being used for the sample rather than the numbers involved. Indeed, Smith and Eatough (2007) warn of the potential problems of data overload when deciding who to include in a sample. The issue here is one of suitability. In phenomenology, the question is whether or not the sample can provide insights and experiences relating to the question at hand so as to enable an in-depth investigation and provide sufficient data for the researchers to interpret.

Usually within phenomenology, sample sizes are small. Numbers vary, though they are generally between 1 and 12, with Smith and Eatough (2007) reporting that, in the case of IPA, the mean is around 8. These are only a guide, however, as all phenomenological approaches warn against having hard or rigid rules (Hallett, 1995). Instead, researchers should be guided by the principles of the questions they wish to study, access to subjects and their ability to appropriately illuminate their experiences, so a single idiographic study may be appropriate. As Silverman (2011) points out, were a qualitative research sample size to be large enough to satisfy generalisability criteria, the researchers would be unable to provide the depth or method of analysis preferred by qualitative investigators. One might argue that researchers' anxieties about providing what they perceive to be valid samples in the eyes of others (their examiners) can override being guided instead by the processes of a qualitative approach.

Ways of collecting data within the phenomenological tradition generally echo those of many qualitative approaches, relying on semi-structured interviews carried out with relatively small numbers of people, chosen for the samples based on their having experience of the subject matter to be studied. The interviews are recorded and, in most instances, last around 45 minutes to an hour in length, though, again, there are no rules regarding how long interviews should be. It is better to be led by the idea that enough time is enough.

Analysis in phenomenology

Streubert and Carpenter (2010: 39) offer a clear and succinct summation of methodological interpretations for researchers considering undertaking a phenomenological study. Of note are Collaizzi's (1978) and Streubert's (1991) methods.

Collaizzi begins with:

- a description of the phenomenon of interest to the researcher
- collection of subjects' descriptions of the phenomenon
- reading of all of the subjects' descriptions of the phenomenon
- returning to the original transcripts and extracting significant statements
- trying to spell out the meanings of each significant statement
- organising the aggregate formalised meanings into a cluster of themes
- writing an exhaustive description
- returning to the subjects for their validation of the description
- if new data are revealed during the validation, incorporating them into an exhaustive description.

Streubert (1991) uses a Husserlian approach to data management in the following way:

- explicating a personal description of the phenomenon of interest
- bracketing the researcher's presuppositions

- interviewing participants in an unfamiliar setting
- carefully reading the transcripts of the interviews to obtain a general sense of participants' experiences
- reviewing the scripts to uncover essences
- apprehending essential relationships
- developing formalised descriptions of phenomena
- returning to participants for them to validate the descriptions
- reviewing the relevant literature
- distributing the findings to the nursing community.

Diekelmann (1992) outlines a seven-step approach to handling hermeneutic analysis:

1. the transcripts are read and reread to obtain a global understanding
2. interpretative analysis is made in the form of summaries for each transcript
3. sample transcripts are sent to two others with cultural knowledge of the phenomena
4. themes are shared and discrepancies dealt with (with recourse to the original recordings) and a composite analysis of each script is written
5. an analysis is made of the texts, incorporating themes from the validation meeting
6. there is further dialogue between validators and researcher to identify a constitutative pattern
7. a rough draft of themes is given to one validator and participant so that unsubstantiated meanings can be removed.

The above demonstrate some similarities and differences, but should not be used as a recipe to be followed slavishly. Instead, each approach shows that different perspectives on the ways in which researchers might use phenomenology can be used to explore meaning and the experiences of others.

CASE STUDY

There are many examples of phenomenological research in healthcare and applied fields. Professor Tom Mason would always begin a lecture on qualitative methods with statistics highlighting phenomenology's pre-eminence in nursing papers, wondering why nurses in particular were drawn to the approach. He would suggest that it is not just a fear of statistics and something about the nature of healthcare work.

In the study outlined below, the researchers represent the fields of nursing and psychology, public health and learning disabilities and used IPA to investigate decisionmaking in evidence-based nursing practice.

Williams et al. (2010) studied 12 intellectual disability nurses, seeking information concerning their decision-making and evidence-based practice when supporting the users of health services. IPA was chosen as it enabled the researchers to adopt the viewpoint of an 'insider, sharing a common language and culture' (Irvine et al., 2008, cited in Williams et al., 2010: 200).

The 12 nurses were individually interviewed by the researchers using a semi-structured format comprised of four sections. In the first section, the respondents were asked to describe an instance of them being responsible for a care episode. The second section led on to a series of open-ended questions focusing on the decision-making processes used by the nurses during the episodes of care reported. The third and fourth sections focused on the nurses' knowledge of evidence-based practice. The interviews were comparatively short, lasting between 22 and 38 minutes and the recordings were transcribed verbatim, though identifying markers were removed from the final copies to ensure anonymity.

The analysis followed Smith and Osborn's (2008) method, the transcripts being read and reread to enable the researchers to familiarise themselves with the data. The process of recording analysis as it emerges in IPA uses a table with three vertical columns, the transcript within the central section, a column to the left for the researchers' responses to the data and initial interpretation arising from the detailed reading and then a column to the right in which to record themes as they emerge. In this process we can see the researchers as insider, as a part of the analysis and also building themes of phenomena. Themes are verified by a process of linking data via the transcripts and creating a master list of themes. Each interview creates a master list, as IPA seeks to establish idiographic understanding before generalising themes.

Although in qualitative research and phenomenology in particular, validity is not sought in the way it is in quantitative studies, the question of dependability or trustworthiness is, nevertheless, central. Coch (1995) describes ensuring that there is an audit trail as means of demonstrating the worthiness of a study. In IPA, Smith and Osborn (2008) rely on a process of independent forward and backward chaining of the data and theme development. They do not advocate returning to the respondents for validation, however, as such comments would form further data, necessitating a further stage of analysis.

Williams et al. (2010) used two supervisors to trail a sample of the transcripts to ensure the validity of the conclusions drawn from the study. One supervisor commenced at the beginning of the process and followed the same steps as the researchers and the other began with the final themes and trailed back to the original transcripts.

CONCLUSION

As stated earlier, work undertaken in phenomenology is determined by a number of factors, not least the ontological position of the researcher. Issues in this form of study focus on differences between epistemological versus philosophical positions. Arguably it is more important that researchers understand that transcendental and interpretative phenomenology are not interchangeable worlds. Each approach brings with it a set of assumptions, starting points and maps that guide and illuminate the world being investigated. Irrespective of how good a study is, the importance of the investigation's congruence will determine its clarity and worth. Whether researchers take Husserl's position of *epoché* or bracketing and separation and seek, via eidetic reduction, to arrive at the essence of an experience or, instead, decide that one's part in the world of research is inescapably joined with that of the subjects and *dasein* or being there is the starting point for discovery of what it means to be is less important than undertaking one approach *or* the other.

Contemporary advantages may be obtained by researchers following an IPA approach. It recognises the benefits of hermeneutics, where meaning and understanding are cocreated, while maintaining a view about the universality of subjects. A compromise maybe, though, when trying to determine a realistic and workable approach to follow, modifying similar yet fundamentally divergent approaches rather than rejecting one in favour of another, appears to have a commonsense ring to it. In addition, a thriving and supportive community of IPA researchers exists on electronic discussion boards and regular conferences are held to help novice phenomenologists begin their studies. An added advantage of IPA is the possibility of contact between the originators of the approach and today's researchers for, unlike Heidegger or Husserl, whose work is mediated via countless translations of their writings and filtered through scholars of differing persuasions, IPA can be sourced from contemporary sources and originators alike.

In the end, researchers will decide what makes sense to them, though what they should not forget is that, more important than ontological or epistemological notions, the question at the heart of an enquiry needs to determine the method, or should do.

FURTHER READING

Streubert, H.J. and Carpenter, D.R. (2010) *Qualitative Research in Nursing: Advancing the humanistic imperative* (5th edn). London: Lippincott, Williams & Wilkins.

REFERENCES

Coch, T. (1995) 'Interpretive approaches in nursing research: The influence of Husserl and Heidegger', *Journal of Advanced Nursing*, 21 (5): 827–36.

Colaizzi, P.F. (1978) 'Psychological research as the phenomenologist views it', in R. Valle, and M. King (eds), *Existential Phenomenological Alternative for Psychology*. New York: Oxford University Press. pp. 58–62.

Crotty, M. (1996) *Phenomenology and Nursing Research*. Melbourne: Churchill Livingstone.

Diekelmann, N.L. (1992) 'Learning-as-testing: A Heideggerian hermeneutical analysis of the lived experience of students and teachers in nursing', *Advanced Nursing Science*, 14 (3): 72–83.

Giorgi, A. (1985) *Phenomenology and Psychological Research*. Pittsburgh, PA: Duquesne University Press.

Hallett, C. (1995) 'Understanding the phenomenological approach to research', *Nurse Researcher*, 3 (5): 55–65.

Holloway, I. and Wheeler, S. (2010) *Qualitative Research in Nursing and Healthcare* (3rd edn). Oxford: Wiley-Blackwell.

Lopez, K.A. and Willis, D.G. (2004) 'Descriptive versus interpretive phenomenology: Their contributions to nursing knowledge', *Qualitative Health Research*, 14 (5): 726–35.

Reid, K., Flowers, P. and Larkin, M. (2005) 'Exploring lived experience', *The Psychologist*, 18 (1): 20–23.

Silverman, D. (2011) *Interpreting Qualitative Data* (4th edn). London: Sage.

Smith, J.A., and Eatough, V. (2007) 'Interpretative phenomenological analysis', in E. Lyons and A.Coyle (eds), *Analysing Qualitative Data in Psychology*. London: Sage. pp. 35–50.

Smith, J.A. and Osborn, M. (2008) 'Interpretative phenomenological analysis', in J.A. Smith (ed.), *Qualitative Psychology: A practical guide to methods*. London: Sage. pp. 53–80.

Smith, J.A., Flowers, P. and Larkin, M. (2009). *Interpretative Phenomenological Analysis: Theory method and research*. London: Sage.

Streubert, H.J. (1991) 'Phenomenologic research as a theoretic initiative in community health nursing', *Public Health Nursing*, 8 (2): 119–23.

Streubert, H.J. and Carpenter, D.R. (2010) *Qualitative Research in Nursing: Advancing the humanistic imperative* (5th edn). London: Lippincott, Williams & Wilkins.

Van Kaam, A. (1969) *Existential Foundations of Psychology*. New York: Image Books.

Walters, A.J. (1995) 'The phenomenological movement: Implications for nursing', *Journal of Advanced Nursing*, 22 (4): 791–9.

Williams, R.W., Roberts, G.W, Irvine, F.E. and Hastings, R.P. (2010) 'Exploring decision making in intellectual disability nursing practice: A qualitative study', *Journal of Intellectual Disabilities*, 14 (3): 197–220.

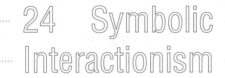

24 Symbolic Interactionism

Robin James Smith

DEFINITION

'Symbolic interactionism' is a sociological tradition that seeks to understand the social world by giving attention to the way meaning, experience and social action are organised in everyday life. A defining assumption is that social definitions and meanings are not static but, rather, produced and modified in human (inter)action. Importantly, once social meanings are established, they come to frame and guide the response of the individual to a given phenomenon, setting or event.

The 'processual', 'reflexive' and 'action-orientated' assumptions of interactionism are grounded in pragmatist philosophy and Weberian interpretivism. The self, and the performances in and through which people accomplish social roles, present themselves to others and react to the performances and actions of others are, thus, central concerns. Such performances are understood within the context of various settings, such as healthcare institutions. Qualitative approaches and, particularly, fieldwork are central to interactionist research.

KEY POINTS

Symbolic interactionism is a term coined by Herbert Blumer, covering a range of approaches. The following are common points of convergence, starting with Blumer's (1969: 2) three key assumptions of interactionism:

- individuals act towards things on the basis of the meanings that the things have for them
- the meaning of such things arises out of the social interactions we have with others
- these meanings are handled in, and modified via, an interpretative process of dealing with the things encountered
- things that come to be defined as real are real in their consequences
- the experience of the individual is contextualised within wider collective practices, social institutions and structures
- interactionism is an empirical approach to the study of social life, using a range of methods, but prioritising participant observation
- interactionist research studies processes, settings and institutions in which individuals and structure are made meaningful in everyday life and, thus, come to have a social presence

DISCUSSION

Symbolic interactionism is a label that glosses over a range of approaches to studying and theorising everyday life. Such variations, many of which are subtle, have common roots in pragmatism, especially that of George Herbert Mead (1934 [1967]) and phenomenology (see Reynolds, 2003).

The tradition can be divided into at least four main 'schools', of which the Chicago School and the Iowa School are perhaps the best known. Only the former is considered here, although it is worth noting that, under the guidance of M.H. Kuhn, the Iowa School developed a positivist strand of interactionism, utilising experiments and quantitative measures in an attempt to provide universal social rules and predictions of social conduct (Meltzer et al., 1975).

While the Iowa School reflected the dominant methodology of the social sciences in America at the time, the work of the various generations of the Chicago School represented a radical break with positivism and structural functionalism. The early research programme of the Chicago School was marked by an empirical approach that prioritised fieldwork as means of studying the complexities of urban society. Robert Park, founding member of the Chicago School, famously, instructed his students to proceed as follows (in an unpublished quote from circa 1925, recorded by Howard Becker, often reproduced):

> Go and sit in the lounges of the luxury hotels and on the doorsteps of the flop houses; sit on the Gold Coast settees and the slum shakedowns; sit in the orchestra hall and in the Star and Garter burlesque. In short, gentlemen, go and get the seat of your pants dirty in real research.

This open-spirited form of enquiry, sensitive to the everyday life of social settings, was consolidated by Blumer (1969) in an elucidation closely following the Meadian emphasis on the emergent nature of the social self, reflexively aware and responsive to that of others, and the constitution of meaning and objects in and via interaction. The insistence on the socially constructed nature of meaning and, therefore, reality does not devolve meaning to mystical, purely subjective or imaginary forces or suggest that 'anything goes'. Rather, interactionism attends to observable processes and material arrangements in which things are defined as real and come to have real, observable consequences.

It follows that Blumer was critical of experimental and survey-based research that fails to access the social meanings framing and determining how individuals respond to objects and situations. For Blumer, the goal and means of social research was to sensitively 'feel one's way' in to the experience of the other, documenting and describing the settings, arrangements and processes that shape the experience of the individual in the context of wider social formations and processes, as realised and negotiated in everyday performances. A requirement, then, is to experience something of the social world of the researched by participating in it for a considerable length of time.

The assumption that situated, local interaction is the locus of socially organised and organising processes finds 'a particular congruence between interactionism and ethnography which goes deeper than a mere preference for "the qualitative"' (Atkinson and Housley, 2000: 120). Interactionist fieldwork draws on a wide range of sources in attempting to produce and gather the 'richest possible data' in order to understand the lived experience of a particular setting or institution (Lofland and Lofland, 1995). Fieldwork enables a sensitive understanding of the conditions, environment and situations that groups and individuals are responding to, negotiating and producing. As summarised by Goffman (1989: 125–6):

> It's one [technique] of getting data ... by subjecting yourself, your own body and your own personality, and your own social situation, to the set of contingencies that play upon a set of individuals, so that you can physically and ecologically penetrate their circle of response to their social situation, or their work situation, or their ethnic situation or whatever. ... To me that's the core of observation. If you don't get yourself in that situation I don't think you can do a piece of serious work. ... You're artificially forcing yourself to be tuned in to something that you then pick up as a witness – not as an interviewer, not as a listener, but as a witness to how they react to what gets done to and around them.

CASE STUDY

Interactionism has contributed much, in both theory and method, to the field of healthcare research. Well-known examples include Roth's (1963) study of a tuberculosis sanatorium (while himself a patient) and Glaser and Strauss' (1965, 1968) work on the 'dying role'. All make a feature of sustained and sensitive fieldwork, detailed description and the production of generalisable concepts that reveal not only the local phenomena in question but also broader aspects of social organisation. There are many such studies from which to choose. Yet, if these are the criteria, Goffman's (1961 [1991]) *Asylums* is a prime candidate.

The essays that comprise *Asylums* develop a description of the 'total institution' – a situation in which the entirety of an individual's experience is managed by an institution (monasteries, army barracks, prisons and, of course, mental asylums are examples). From his position working as an assistant in St Elizabeth's Hospital, Washington DC, Goffman documented life in the asylum – its routines, official and unofficial systems, hierarchies and the processes by means of which 'inmates' identities are (re)formed following the stripping away of their existing means of performing and understanding themselves (what Goffman called the 'mortification of the Self'). Importantly, the description came from the perspective of the patients. One essay describes the ways in which 'inpatients' are subjected to a range of 'people processing' procedures, revealing 'the limited extent to which a conception of one's Self can be sustained when the usual setting of supports for it are suddenly removed' (Goffman, 1961 [1991]: 137). This is followed by an incredibly detailed examination of the means by which the patients managed to preserve a sense of Self – by securing personal space, covert channels of communication and various methods of 'working the system'.

Goffman's interest in such extreme institutional arrangements lay also in a concern with the structure, frailty and resilience of the Self in American society. An aim of the work was to challenge perceptions of mental illness and 'deviant' behaviour by illustrating how patients and staff alike develop social worlds that appear normal, once viewed through their eyes.

Goffman employed a form of comparative analysis, not simply selecting a hospital or setting in another country or operating under a different policy regime, but identifying other settings in which the *concept* being explored might be found. *Asylums* is replete with surprising examples, commonalties found in unusual juxtapositions, which expose that which we take for granted, revealing its socially constructed origins.

Goffman also developed a neutral conceptual language to talk about the, often shocking, conditions of the asylum and the behaviours of patients (Becker, 2003). It succeeded in demonstrating how patients' responses to the mortifying process and their negotiation of the 'privilege system' were rational and how we routinely take the position and practices of the privileged and 'experts', such as doctors and consultants, for granted. In this sense, Goffman's (sometimes painfully) detailed, ethnography of life in the asylum is never only about the asylum but, rather, also seeks to generate an understanding and, indeed, new perspective, on the way in which the Self is threatened, reconstituted and preserved by social actors in extremis. By pointing the finger back at wider society (that is, us), *Asylums* did much to change both public and professional perceptions and it is, perhaps, the greatest credit to Goffman that his study is considered a piece of healthcare research rather than a study of social deviance, mental illness and abnormality.

CONCLUSION

Symbolic interactionism contributes a great deal towards understanding how healthcare settings are experienced and socially organised. Direct observation of the workings of hospital wards, GP surgeries and any number of specialist clinics enables a sensitivity to the experiences of people who have business there in ways that contrived means (such as interviews) do not. Interactionism is, of course, more than a directive to fieldwork. Fieldwork – situated, local, mundane – within an interactionist framework should also develop concepts that advance an under-standing of generic social processes, applicable across a range of settings and institutions.

Interactionist-inspired studies of healthcare settings and institutions thus find, in the local, the (re)production of generic orders of action and interaction, prac-tices and rituals, systems and processes that connect the part to the whole (Atkinson et al., 2008). In documenting and describing the workings of everyday situations where 'well-placed people ... give official imprint to versions reality' (Goffman, 1982), interactionist research demonstrates the *social* foundations of such relations and, in so doing, highlights the cracks where possibilities for change might lie.

FURTHER READING

Charmaz and Olesen (2003) – see reference below – provide an accessible overview of interac-tionist contributions to the field and, especially, the view of healthcare and medicine as social institution. The handbook of which the chapter is part provides an excellent general point of reference for interactionism. You should also read one of the many ethnographic monographs. If you were to pick just one, Glaser and Strauss' *Awareness of Dying* represents the points covered in this chapter well.

Charmaz, K. and Olesen, V. (2003) 'Medical Institutions', in L.T. Reynolds and N.J. Herman-Kinney (eds), *Handbook of Symbolic Interactionism*. Oxford: Alta Mira Press. pp. 637–56.

REFERENCES

Atkinson, P. and Housley, W. (2000) *Interactionism*. London: Sage.

Atkinson, P., Delamont, S. and Housley, W. (2008) *Contours of Culture: Complex ethnography and the ethnography of complexity*. Lanham, MD: AltaMira Press.

Becker, H. (2003) 'The politics of presentation: Goffman and total institutions', *Symbolic Interaction*, 26 (4): 659–69.

Blumer, H. (1969) *Symbolic Interactionism: Perspective and method*. Englewood Cliffs, NJ: Prentice Hall.

Glaser, B. and Strauss, A. (1965) *Awareness of Dying*. Chicago, IL: Aldine.

Glaser, B. and Strauss, A. (1968) *Time for Dying*. Chicago, IL: Aldine.

Goffman, E. (1961 [1991]) *Asylums*. London: Penguin.

Goffman, E. (1982) 'Presidential address', *American Sociological Review*, 48: 1–17.

Goffman, E. (1989) 'On fieldwork', *Journal of Contemporary Ethnography*, 18 (2): 123–32.

Lofland and Lofland (1995) *Analyzing Social Settings: A guide to qualitative observation and analy-sis*. Belmont, CA: Wadsworth.

Mead, G.H. (1934 [1967]) *Mind, Self and Society*. Chicago, IL: University of Chicago Press.

Meltzer, B.N., Petras, J.W. and Reynolds, L.T. (1975) *Symbolic Interactionism: Genesis, varieties and criticism.* London: Routledge & Kegan Paul.

Reynolds, L.T. (2003) 'Intellectual precursors', in L.T. Reynolds and N.J. Herman-Kinney *Handbook of Symbolic Interactionism.* Lanham, MD: AltaMira Press. pp. 39–58.

Roth, J.A. (1963) *Timetables.* New York: Bobbs-Merrill.

25   Vignette Research

Dave Mercer

DEFINITION

'Vignettes' are used by researchers working in both quantitative and qualitative paradigms, but the focus in this chapter is on their function as an adaptable aid to exploring ideas, attitudes and values as they are expressed in the language of research respondents. In this context, vignettes are simulations of real events that provide a 'key' to elicit talk in interview situations. They can be produced in different media forms and are often employed when the topics under discussion are of a sensitive nature.

KEY POINTS

Vignettes are:

- A versatile and flexible adjunct to interviews with individuals or as part of focus group and other qualitative research
- A way of addressing sensitive topics where observation is not possible
- A cost-effective technique when funding and time are limited
- A component of multi-method and multi-modal research designs

DISCUSSION

Credible qualitative research relies on rich data and rigorous analysis. This chapter focuses on the former and discusses how vignettes can provide an imaginative methodological resource in the process of data collection.

The vignette is a tool used in social science research and has a long history in disciplines such as anthropology and psychology. Though early nursing studies recognised the usefulness of the vignette (Wilson and While, 1998), it is only more recently that it has received significant attention. Indeed, most textbooks on nursing and healthcare research make little, if any, reference to the vignette in their content or index lists. It is, however, well defined by Bloor and Wood (2006: 183) as 'a technique used in structured and in-depth interviews as well as focus groups, providing sketches of fictional (or fictionalised) scenarios'. As a way of accessing ideas, attitudes and values, participants are invited to respond to these by using them as a means of reflecting on, and drawing from, personal experience.

Traditionally, vignettes have been short pieces of text, such as an abbreviated case study. Over time and with technological advances, however, vignette methodology has evolved to embrace other formats and media than the written word. There are vignettes in the form of images, such as cartoons, video recordings or live events – the aims of the studies shaping their design (Hughes and Huby, 2002).

A vignette can be introduced in a face-to-face meeting or via a computer. In research projects where participants are required to comment on sensitive or intimate aspects of their lives, vignettes have proved particularly useful. Because the respondent can assume the 'identity' of a fictional character, the vignette's content mediates discussion and places a distance between the speakers and the events they are prepared to share with the researchers. It is suggested that this protective mechanism enhances the quality of the data, because the interviewees are more likely to talk about subjects that could, otherwise, cause embarrassment or lead to them closing up. By 'desensitising' the issues, they become 'less personal' and, therefore, 'less threatening' (Wilks, 2004). This advantage of vignettes also relates, closely, to safeguarding subjects in an ethical sense. Vignettes can be designed to cover topics which cannot be observed in the natural world, such as sexual abuse, and used when questionnaires and self-report studies run the risk of generating socially appropriate responses.

In the context of research philosophy and design, the vignette complements debates about the constructive nature of knowledge, which occupy a pivotal place in qualitative enquiry (Potter and Wetherell, 1987). In such studies, discourse analysis is recommended as a strategy to explore contradictions and dilemmas, looking at the performative functions of language when constructing versions of the 'Self', negotiating 'identity' and reconciling tensions in the social world. The vignette provides an entry point to the complexity of talk and furnishes an interesting perspective on how health or social care researchers might explore interpretative repertoires that discursively construct their respective fields of practice and moral decisionmaking (Wilks, 2004), leading to a better understanding of relations between 'values' and 'actions'. Similarly, from a phenomenological perspective, where vignettes capture the lived-experience of respondents, as Jenkins and colleagues (2010) discuss, they can be used to explore *group values* rather than predict *individual behaviours*. To understand longitudinal attitude changes, they recommend using 'developmental' rather than 'snapshot' vignettes.

Finally, a note of caution needs to be introduced to the discussion regarding what have been identified as shortcomings or pitfalls of the vignette as a research tool. One theoretical issue is the potential dissonance between 'real-life' processes and 'vignette scenarios' (Hughes and Huby, 2002), calling for a close correspondence between vignette content and respondents' experiences.

A related critique is the artificiality of the exercise and extent to which vignettes can embrace the complexity and nuances of social life. These concerns are sustainable, but it needs to be remembered that no research design is 'foolproof' and the ideas discussed in this chapter suggest one technique among many that can be used to move social researchers closer to the social world of those they seek to engage.

CASE STUDY

This short case study outlines a collegiate initiative to explore and understand the relations between institutional culture and care planning in one high-security forensic setting. These large hospitals provide treatment for disordered offenders, the role of the nurses being a hybrid mix of therapeutic engagement and custodial containment. A significant number of the patient population are deemed extremely dangerous and spend many years in an insular environment where the ultimate goal is rehabilitation rather than punishment.

The researchers sought to critically interrogate how nursing staff constructed care plans for individuals who were defined in terms of both their criminal behaviour (such as rape) and mental disorders (such as psychopathy). The findings have been discussed elsewhere (Richman et al., 1999), so the aim here is to look at how a series of vignettes that acted as a prompt for the respondents' talk complemented the philosophical design of the study.

The research question was rooted firmly in the clinical environment of the ward, where formal and informal nurse–patient interactions occurred and centred on the challenge that faced forensic nurses translating broader nursing theories into a unique healthcare setting defined by medicalised crime.

Intellectually, the project had been inspired by an interest in social constructionism and discursive practice (Burr, 2003). In other words, the function of collective language as shared words, symbols and values in texturing the social space of the ward and constructing the object/subject of their attentions. It became necessary, therefore, to capture the various discourses that the nurses drew on to explain offending, offenders and treatment. At this point in time, no training had been given to ward-based staff in terms of applying a bio-medical model of intervention to men who were commonly referred to as 'mad and bad' (Prins, 1994). In this sense, the study brought nursing practice under the lens of critical sociological investigation in a way that, at the time, might contribute to the development of an embryonic branch of the profession.

It had been decided to use in-depth, semi-structured, interviews to collect data from those nurses who agreed to participate in the study. Gaining ethical approval to undertake this work was only the start in terms of entering a field notable for its sinister and secretive history (Pilgrim, 2007). A strategy was needed to encourage respondents to talk openly and candidly about issues that Lee (1993) describes as 'sensitive topics', while maintaining an emotionally safe 'distance' (Finch, 1987). The vignette proved to be of great value, representing a 'bridge' between the macro-level disciplinary technology of forensic psychiatry and the micro-level discourses of those who operate as its 'frontline' agents.

Table 25.1   Axial principles of the construction of vignettes (adapted from Richman and Mercer, 2002)

Vignette A: Abuse and physical injury resulting in the death of a one-year-old child.

Vignette B: Recidivist, violent, rape where the victims were elderly women.

Vignette C: Abduction, sexual assault and murder of a nine-year-old boy.

Vignette D: Sadistic and ritualised behaviours in the childhood of a spousal murderer.

Vignette E: Killing of a stranger where the offender heard instructional voices.

Vignette F: A fatal attack where the offender believed he or she was persecuted by 'aliens'.

The research team developed a series of six short vignettes (A–F), each approximately 250 words in length. These were printed on A4 paper, in an accessible font size, to make reading them while talking easier. The content of each vignette sketched out the case history of one offender–patient who closely resembled the offence patterns of detained men at the study site. All of the details provided in the vignettes were adapted and anonymised cases from the professional literature. This meant they would have resonance for respondents, triggering comparisons, while avoiding the need to discuss actual patients in their care. The construction of individual vignettes was hinged to an axial principle (see Table 25.1), but efforts were made to remove clinical–psychiatric linguistic signifiers, such as diagnostic language. For each vignette, two versions were produced, with the offender described as 'black' or 'white', to consider ethnicity as a possible variant in the construction of accounts. One vignette (A) concerned a female perpetrator, to explore gendered discourse, though the hospital population was all male.

The research interviews lasted between 45 minutes and 2 hours and took place in quiet rooms, when staff were available to participate. Respondents were given copies of the vignettes that they read and commented on. They self-selected those of particular interest, providing the opportunity to generate co-constructed accounts via reflection and dialogue (Kvale, 1996), the vignettes acting as 'keys' to unlock the discourse of forensic wards.

During the interviews, researchers picked up on cues and used exploratory prompts to focus on five key themes that guided the collection of data:

1. nurses' perceptions of different types of offence
2. nurses' perceptions of relations between mental health and offending
3. nurses' use of theoretical and non-theoretical explanations
4. nurses' use of language in relation to ethnicity and gender
5. nurses' talk about care planning and treatment issues for disordered offenders.

CONCLUSION

Though brief, this chapter will hopefully kindle the interest of those looking for different ways to approach, and enrich, qualitative research data collection. Though overlooked by most mainstream textbooks, the vignette has a long and respected history in social science. Each one can be both complex and simple in its construction and application, but all offer a versatile tool, particularly when faced with budgetary limitations, time constraints or sensitive topic areas. They can be used alone or as part of multi-method approaches.

FURTHER READING

Barter, C. and Renold, E. (2000) '"I wanna tell you a story": exploring the application of vignettes in qualitative research with children and young people', *International Journal of Social Research Methodology*, 3: 307–23.

Bondani, M.A., MacEntee, M.I., Ross Bryant, S. and O'Neill, B. (2008) 'Using written vignettes in focus groups to discuss oral health as a sensitive topic', *Qualitative Health Research*, 18: 1145–53.

Hughes, R. (1998) 'Considering the vignette technique and its application to a study of drug injecting and HIV risk and safer behaviour', *Sociology of Health and Illness*, 20: 381–400.

Merry, L., Clausen, C., Cagnon, A.J., Carnevale, F., Jeannotte, J., Saucier, J. and Oxman-Martinez, J. (2011) 'Improving qualitative interviews with newly arrived migrant women', *Qualitative Health Research*, 21: 976–86.

Schoenberg, N.E. and Ravdal, H. (2000) 'Using vignettes in awareness and attitudinal research', *International Journal of Social Research Methodology*, 3: 63–74.

REFERENCES

Bloor, M. and Wood, F. (2006) *Keywords in Qualitative Methods: A vocabulary of research concepts*. London: Sage.

Burr, V. (2003) *Social Constructionism* (2nd edn). Abingdon: Routledge.

Finch, J. (1987) 'The vignette technique in survey research', *Sociology*, 21: 105–14.

Hughes, R. and Huby, M. (2002) 'The application of vignettes in social and nursing research' *Journal of Advanced Nursing*, 37: 382–6.

Jenkins, N., Bloor, M., Fischer, J., Berney, L. and Neale, J. (2010) 'Putting it in context: The use of vignettes in qualitative interviewing', *Qualitative Research*, 10: 175–98.

Kvale, S. (1996) *InterViews: An introduction to qualitative research interviewing*. London: Sage.

Lee, R. (1993) *Doing Research on Sensitive Topics*. London: Sage.

Pilgrim, D. (ed.) (2007) *Inside Ashworth: Professional reflections of institutional life*. Oxford: Radcliffe.

Potter, J. and Wetherell, M. (1987) *Discourse and Social Psychology: Beyond attitudes and behaviour*. London: Sage.

Prins, H. (1994) 'Psychiatry and the concept of evil: Sick in heart or sick in mind?', *British Journal of Psychiatry*, 165: 297–302.

Richman, J. and Mercer, D. (2002) 'The vignette revisited: Evil and the forensic nurse', *Nurse Researcher*, 9 (4): 70–82.

Richman, J., Mercer, D, and Mason, T. (1999) 'The social construction of evil in a forensic setting', *Journal of Forensic Psychiatry*, 10: 300–308.

Wilks, T. (2004) 'The use of vignettes in qualitative research', *Qualitative Social Work*, 3: 78–87.

Wilson, J. and While, A.E. (1998) 'Methodological issues surrounding the use of vignettes in qualitative research', *Journal of Interprofessional Care*, 12: 79–86.

ACKNOWLEDGEMENTS

The enquiring and intellectual spirit of much-missed friends – Professor Joel Richman and Professor Tom Mason.

key concepts in nursing and healthcare research

Jan Woodhouse

DEFINITION

'Visual research' or methodology involves utilising an image. The image may be part of the data or it can be used as a prompt for discussion.

Visual materials, according to Rose (2007), are representations of the ways in which people behave in everyday life. Gilroy (2006) points out that a picture, such as a drawing, can promote a research question and may be psychologically revealing. Traditionally, this form of research has been used in ethnographic studies (Pink, 2006), but it can now be found in a variety of disciplines, such as art therapy, media, education, environmental studies and healthcare and social care (Emmison and Smith, 2000; Gilroy, 2006; Woodhouse, 2012).

Visual data can be in the form of fine art, still images, such as book illustrations, maps, postcards, photographs, paintings and cartoons, advertising, signage, or moving images, such as films, video and TV programmes (Emmison and Smith, 2000; Rose, 2007).

KEY POINTS

- Visual methods can be used in either quantitative or qualitative paradigms
- There is a range of research traditions to choose from
- There are advantages and disadvantages to consider when using the approach
- There are specific ethical dimensions to visual methods that need to be considered
- There is specific terminology connected to visual methods, which helps when analysing the data
- Visual methods can benefit from rigour, validity and reliability

DISCUSSION

Visual methodology and research paradigms

Visual methodology can fit into either qualitative or quantitative paradigms. As with any research, the methodology is dependent on the question being asked. In 2006, Pink, for example, used visual ethnography (a qualitative approach), in the form of photographs, to explore the lives of people in different cultures, but a similar approach has also been used in a hospital setting in order to map a patient's journey through its services (Woodhouse, 2012). In hospitals, photography has been used to consider how the operating theatre functions and a video camera utilised in an intensive care unit to record power relationships of clinicians and staff. Also, archival data, in the form of postcards (a quantitative approach) and published cartoons, have been used to explore the changing image of nurses and investigate gender issues related to patient participations (Woodhouse, 2012).

Using drawings was an approach taken by Dumont (2008) to explore children's family relationships, which were mapped out using differing colours to determine the strength of the relationship. Similarly, another study used drawings by individual student nurses to explore their perceptions of what ageing might do to them (Woodhouse, 2012).

The variety of traditions within visual methodology

There are, along with differing forms of data, also differing approaches to the point at which participants and researchers interact. Cousin (2009) categorises them according to the subject, media type, research setting and intention or context of the research, as shown in Table 26.1.

Similarly, Wagner (2011) notes six methods of enquiry:

- artefact acquisition and analysis
- photo and video documentation
- researcher-guided image elicitation
- image-based ethnography
- neuro-physical measurements of visual perception
- formal and semiotic analyses of visual representations.

Table 26.1 Visual research traditions

Category	Subject	Media	Setting	Intention
Archival data	None	Films, photographs, art, advertisements	Thematic	Visual supports the research activity
Visual ethnography	Observed overtly or covertly	Film, video or photographs taken	Research setting	Visual supports the research activity
Visual as prompt	Shown visual Data, such as photographs	Film, photographs, drawings	Not specific	Visual chosen to direct discussion
Visual elicitation	Chooses own archival material	Photographs, postcards, posters, pictures, video	Not specific	Visual directs the research activity
Auto-driven visual elicitation	Take photographs or video	Photographs, video	Research setting or thematic	Visual directs the research activity
Picture elicitation (or externally driven visual elicitation)	Draw a picture	Drawings, paintings	Not specific	Visual supports the research activity
Video diaries	Records reflective accounts	Video	Research setting	Visual can direct or support the research activity

Emmison and Smith (2000) also comment on the different modes of the images, classifying them into the 'scientific mode' and the 'narrative mode'. The notion of the scientific mode is a familiar one in the sphere of nursing where, for example, a wound might be photographed, but it can also be used by asking participants to take a photograph on a topic or perhaps as part of a visual diary. The scientific mode is an image that becomes a moment frozen in time. A drawing may also be utilised in this way. The alternative is the narrative mode, which is a series of photographs or images that record an event.

Advantages and disadvantages

When choosing visual methodology as a research approach, there has to be a weighing up of its advantages and disadvantages (Woodhouse, 2012). In terms of the advantages, they are that:

- there is a lot of material already available via the Internet, magazines and other sources
- data can be obtained quickly as digital cameras can easily take photographs and/or record drawings or paintings (Mitchell, 2011)
- electronic copies are easy to store and collate
- software enables you to focus on particular aspects of a photograph, zooming in on a particular object, or example
- crucially, research is *with* informants rather than *on* them.

Its disadvantages are that:

- issues may arise involving how to use technology (Mitchell, 2011)
- you need to gain permission, which might be problematic (photographs especially can show up good and bad aspects of an environment)
- if participants are photographed, they may not like their image and seek to withdraw the photo from the data (Rose, 2007)
- images on their own may not be sufficient – they need to be contextualised.

In addition, there may be copyright issues. For example, simply giving someone a camera to take photos may open up a copyright debate as the photos then belong to 'the photographer' rather than the owner of the camera. Permission to use the photographs produced therefore have to be negotiated with the participants (Rose, 2007). Taking your own photographs may help to overcome this issue, but may not solve the research question if the intention is to gain a participants' eye view of the world. Similarly, if someone produces an artwork, then they need to give permission to have it photographed for research purposes (Gilroy, 2006). Note that it is better to have that permission in writing, rather than verbally. Finally, dissemination may be more problematic as journals and books are reluctant to print images because of the cost. This can be overcome if the journal is an online one, however, where it is easier to publish visual material.

Ethical aspects of the methodology

Any researcher should have an awareness of the ethical principles in research, as has been discussed elsewhere in this book. Rose (2007), however, reminds us that visual methodology researchers should pay specific attention to gaining permission for access to locations where it is planned that images may be taken. Given that data may be captured via the use of cameras or video, then there is an extra dimension to ensuring that the participants are happy with their recorded images, as noted above. If they are unhappy, then the images may have to be blurred to preserve their anonymity (Rose, 2007).

As with any aspect of research, the ethical dimension of collecting, storing and using any data, as well as attending to protecting participants, should not be ignored. In this respect, visual methodology is no different from other forms of data collection.

Analysis of the data

In order to carry out any kind of analysis, researchers need to be aware of the distinct terminology associated with visual methodology as this may guide their route to analysis (see Table 26. 2, which, though not exhaustive, includes the most commonly used terms).

Hence, analysis of an image may depend on the chosen paradigm, the visual data collected and the subsequent level of analysis chosen by the researcher. It is possible to codify aspects of an image in order to arrive at quantitative outcomes. Similarly, a narrative may be sought in order to arrive at meaning for those using a qualitative framework. In other words, the image alone may not be enough. This may be why the use of visual methodology has been quite slow to take off as an academic discipline, as there is a need for supplementary data. Nevertheless, it can hold its place in the research process because of its adaptability.

The rigour, validity and reliability of visual methods

As with any research method, the rigour, validity and reliability of the approach should be considered by researchers. As visual methodology is a relative newcomer to the academic world of research, particular attention needs to be paid to these aspects if it is to be accepted. Indeed, Newberry (2011: 662) reminds us, 'Visual scholarship demands that we treat images with the same seriousness and rigour as we apply to other materials with which we work.' Proving attention has been paid to the research question, the chosen approach and the data analysis means the work can be defended. The more visual methods are used, the more rigorous the approach will become, adding to the perception of its validity and reliability.

CASE STUDY

A group of student nurses were asked to draw pictures to show how they relieved their stress. Various genres appeared, such as music, exercise, alcohol, bathing and social circle activities. While the drawings on their own enabled a certain amount

Table 26.2 Some terms used in visual methodology

Term	Meaning	Example
Frame What is the context of the image?	A 'visual device that can create degrees of connection or disconnection between all elements of a composition' (Van Leewen, 2011: 561)	It is the difference between taking a photograph of a landscape and a close-up of a flower in the foreground
Decoding What is the 'preferred', 'hegemonic' or 'dominant' (as intended by the author) meaning that prevails?	Using previously learned (which may be culturally bound) cognitive functions that enable the decoding of a symbolic meaning within an image	A person drawn with a walking stick may indicate age and infirmity
Signs, signifiers, signified	A sign is a thing plus meaning (Rose, 2007), made up of two parts – the signified (a concept of object) and signifier (a sound, image or written word)	A caring person (concept) is signified by an image of a nurse (signifier)
Binary opposites	A simple aspect of analysis – absences may reveal cultural taboos or norms	Man/woman, light/dark, up/down, left/right
Genre	Commonly associated with film and television, but may be used to classify elements in a still image	Drama, romance, children, adults, landscape
Visual semiotics	Layering of meaning using denotation ('What, or who, is being depicted?') and connotation ('What ideas and values are being expressed via what is represented and the way in which it is being represented?') (Van Leewen, 2011)	Fire escape signs, traffic signs, posters, diagrams
Iconography	A shared understanding of what an image can represent	Che Guevara = rebellion Eiffel Tower = Paris/all things French
Symbolism	An image that may hold a personal representation of a concept	A snake = a potent force; a fear; lowly; suppleness; or something else
Diagrammatic and embodied images	Found in drawings and paintings – a diagrammatic image is representational and intentional, an embodied image one in which the meaning emerges after finishing the work (Schaverin, 1999)	A picture of a house and tree may be diagrammatic. The same image, not intentionally drawn, may represent a memory of childhood

of analysis to be carried out – that is, the categorisation of the genres – it was beneficial to ask the students to explain their drawings, too. This enabled researchers to correctly attribute images. For example, instead of an image of someone swimming being categorised as belonging to the exercise genre, after speaking with the student nurse who drew it, it was placed instead in the 'wash it away' category (one supplied by the students) along with other images of baths and bathing. This shows the level of participation that can occur in visual methodology.

CONCLUSION

The use of visual methodology is gaining ground as an accepted form of research in the field of health and social care. It offers a wide range of data-collection formats, which are often readily available to researchers. An understanding, however, of the traditions and terminology of visual research is essential preparation for any researcher considering or choosing this method. There are methods of data analysis in visual methodology that have already been accepted and, as its use expands and a greater body of literature builds, it is expected that others will emerge.

FURTHER READING

Margolis, E. and Pauwels, L. (eds) (2011) *The Sage Handbook of Visual Research Methods*. London: Sage.

Van Leewen, T. and Jewitt, C. (eds) (2001) *Handbook of Visual Analysis*. London: Sage.

REFERENCES

Cousin, G. (2009) *Researching Learning in Higher Education: An introduction to contemporary methods and approaches*. Abingdon: Routledge.

Dumont, R.H. (2008) 'Drawing a family map: An experiential tool for engaging children in family therapy', *Journal of Family Therapy*, 30: 247–59.

Emmison, M. and Smith, P. (2000) *Researching the Visual*. London: Sage.

Gilroy, A. (2006) *Art Therapy, Research and Evidence-based Practice*. London: Sage.

Mitchell, C. (2011) *Doing Visual Research*. London: Sage.

Newberry, D. (2011) 'Making arguments with images: Visual scholarship and academic publishing', in E. Margolis and L. Pauwels (eds), *The Sage Handbook of Visual Research Methods*. London: Sage. pp. 651–64.

Pink, S. (2006) *Doing Visual Ethnography*. London: Sage.

Rose, G. (2007) *Visual Methodologies: An Introduction to the Interpretation of Visual Materials* (2nd edn). London: Sage.

Schaverin, J. (1999) *The Revealing Image*. London: Jessica Kingsley.

Van Leewen, T. (2011) 'Multimodality and multimodal research', in E. Margolis and L. Pauwels (eds), *The Sage Handbook of Visual Research Methods*. London: Sage. pp. 549–69.

Wagner, J. (2011) 'Visual studies and empirical social enquiry', in E. Margolis and L. Pauwels (eds), *The Sage Handbook of Visual Research Methods*. London: Sage. pp. 49–71.

Woodhouse, J. (2012) 'The use of visual methodology in nursing', *Nurse Researcher*, 19 (3): 20–25.

key concepts in nursing and healthcare research

Part 3
Quantitative Research Methods

27 Experimental Design

Roger Watson

DEFINITION

Experimental research is designed to help researchers compare and arbitrate between conflicting hypotheses (see http://explorable.com/experimental-research for detailed information).

KEY POINTS

The key points associated with experimental research are:

- Hypotheses
- Manipulation
- Variables
- Control
- Measurement
- Inferential statistics
- Experimental designs

Hypothesis: an **hypothesis** is a statement of the relationship between two variables that can be tested.

Manipulation: an experiment requires manipulation – something has to be done that enables hypotheses to be compared.

Variables: variables can be independent and dependent; **independent variables** are ones that cannot be changed by the ones you are measuring and **dependent variables** are ones that depend on the independent variables and which are measured in an experiment (http://nces.ed.gov/nceskids/help/user_guide/graph/variables.asp).

Measurement: in experimental research the variables must be capable of measurement using **reliable** and **valid** methods.

Control: there must some means of comparing the hypotheses and this is achieved by control.

Inferential statistics: formal and unbiased comparison of hypotheses can only be made using **inferential statistics.**

Experimental designs: are those where the researcher intervenes in the study to see what effect that intervention has.

DISCUSSION

Hypotheses

An 'hypothesis' is a statement of the relationship between two variables – for example, 'Nursing intervention A is better than nursing intervention B at changing condition X'. Its purpose is to provide an outcome from a piece of quantitative research that can be formally tested using 'inferential statistics'. In experimental research the hypothesis must be about comparing one thing with another using one of a range of the designs described below.

Hypotheses are not unique to experimental research, however, and can be more speculative, such as, 'There will be a relationship between nursing intervention A and condition B'.

Manipulation

In an experiment, the variable of interest is 'manipulated' while the remainder are kept constant or randomly allocated in order that the effect of manipulating the variable of interest can be seen (www.biology-online.org). 'Manipulation' could mean providing a nursing intervention to one group and withholding it from another to see the effect of that intervention.

Control

In an experiment, a 'control' group is one for which the intervention – applied to the intervention group – is not applied to them in order that the two groups can be compared (www.biology-online.org) to see what, if any, effect the intervention has.

Measurement

Experiments involve 'measurement' of the dependent variables in both the intervention and the control groups in order that they can be compared.

Inferential statistics

'Inferential statistics' is the branch of statistics whereby hypothesised relationships between variables can be tested using probability. A commonly applied test in experiments is the 't-test' (see Chapter 33).

Experimental designs

Experimental designs fall into two main categories:

- true experiments
- quasi-experiments (see www.researchconnections.org/childcare/datamethods/experimentsquasi.jsp for more on these).

A 'true experiment' is very specific, describing a situation in which researchers manipulate the independent variables of the experiment – the intervention – to effect a change in the dependent variable(s). In addition, in a true experiment, there will be a control group and random allocation of participants to the control group and the group receiving the intervention. Randomly allocating participants in this way guards against 'bias' – that is, the researchers possibly introducing factors into the experiment that would favour a particular outcome. 'Random allocation' means that potential participants are allocated to the intervention and control groups at random. This can be achieved by using sets of random numbers for participants, which can be generated by computer. In this way, the researchers do not bias the results of the study and any uncontrollable variables are randomly distributed between the groups. Bias may be introduced if, for example, researchers deliberately allocate all of the people who are less ill to the treatment group of a study of a drug meant to cure them and all of the sick people to the control group.

The most rigorous experimental design involving human participants is the 'randomised double-blind controlled trial' (RCT). 'Blind', in the context of an experiment, means that either participants in the trial do now know which group they have been allocated to or the researchers do not know and 'double-blind' means that neither know. This is done to minimise the 'placebo effect', which is when participants appear to respond to an intervention whether they have had it or not, simply as a result of having been involved in the trial. When researchers are 'blind' in this way, by using the random numbers for participants rather than their names and so on, it prevents the possibility of the results being manipulated in any way to achieve a favourable outcome.

A 'quasi-experiment' is, broadly, one in which the aspects of manipulation, random allocation or control are relaxed. For example, in the absence of a control group, people may act as their own controls. In a pre-test–post-test design, for example, there would be no intervention for a period, followed by introducing the intervention and then the before and after measurements of the dependent variable would be compared. Alternatively, in situations where it is impossible to allocate the intervention randomly, groups that have either already received or not received the intervention could be compared.

There are many variations on the quasi-experiment and, in many situations, they are perfectly acceptable for practical or ethical reasons. They are, however, never as rigorous as a true experiment.

Additional points

CONSORT (www.consort-statement.org) is an organisation that exists to help with the proper reporting of clinical trials. It is well worth taking a look at its website.

'Intention to treat analysis' is a 'method of analysing results of a randomised controlled trial that includes in the analysis all those cases that should have received a treatment regimen but for whatever reason did not. All cases allocated to each arm of the trial are analysed together as representing that treatment arm, regardless of whether they received or completed the prescribed regimen' (www.medilexicon.com/medicaldictionary.php).

CASE STUDY

The case study described looked at the difficulty older people with dementia have feeding themselves. This difficulty arises because, as dementia progresses, there is an almost inevitable decline in the ability to feed oneself (Watson and Green,

2006). This is associated with weight loss and emaciation, which is distressing for carers and relatives of older people with dementia.

A review of the literature in this area showed that there is no good evidence to support any particular interventions and studies in the area are very poor in terms of design (Watson and Green, 2006). Since the review, some work has been conducted into methods for retraining older people with dementia based on educational methods used with children (Montessori method) and children with learning difficulties (spaced retrieval). These methods have been tested using what is described as 'a single evaluator, blind, and randomised control trial' (Lin et al., 2010) and in a crossover experiment (Lin et al., 2011). The former is described here.

Describing the trial as 'single evaluator, blind, and randomised control' means that the data collection was carried out by single data collectors and not having more than one person to check the collection of data. The data collectors, however, were trained in the use of the assessment instruments. The trial was blind (or single blind) in that the data collectors were unaware of which group (Montessori, spaced retrieval or control) the participants belonged to. The trial was randomised because the participants were randomly allocated to the three groups.

The statistical analysis of the data was complex and beyond the scope of this chapter (a linear mixed model was used), but save to say it was applied to a range of outcomes, including feeding difficulty (Lin et al., 2008), body mass index and the Mini Nutritional Assessment (MNA).

The outcome of the trial was that levels of feeding difficulty in both of the intervention groups declined and the MNA status of the spaced retrieval group improved – both these results were statistically significant. There was no significant difference between intervention and control groups in terms of body mass index.

CONCLUSION

Experiments are designed to test the effectiveness of interventions. There is a range of designs and the most rigorous is the double-blind randomised controlled trial. The outcomes of experiments require the use of statistics to analyse the results.

FURTHER READING

Parahoo, A.K. (2006) *Nursing Research: Principles, process and issues* (2nd edn). Houndmills, Basingstoke: Palgrave Macmillan.
Watson, R., McKenna, H., Cowman, S. and Keady, J. (2008) *Nursing Research: Design and methods*. Edinburgh: Elsevier.

REFERENCES

Lin, L.-C., Huang, Y.-J., Su, S.-G., Watson, R., Tsai, B.W.-J. and Wu, S.-C. (2010) 'Using spaced retrieval and Montessori-based activities in improving eating ability for residents with dementia', *International Journal of Geriatric Psychiatry*, 25: 953–9.
Lin, L.-C., Huang, Y.-J., Watson, R., Wu, S.-C., Lee, Y.-C. and Chou, Y.-C. (2011) 'Using a Montessori method to increase eating ability for institutionalised residents with dementia: A crossover study', *Journal of Clinical Nursing*, 20: 3092–3101.

Lin, L.-C., Watson, R., Lee, Y.-C., Chou, Y.-C. and Wu, S.-C. (2008) 'Edinburgh Feeding Evaluation
    in Dementia (EdFED) scale: Cross-cultural validation of the Chinese version', *Journal of
    Advanced Nursing*, 62, 116–23.
Watson, R. and Green, S. (2006) 'Feeding and dementia: A systematic literature review', *Journal
    of Advanced Nursing*, 54: 86–93.

28 / Quasi-Experimental Design

Vimal Kumar Sharma and Nikhil Sharma

DEFINITION

'Quasi-experimental design' is a research method used to make apparent any difference made by an intervention (effect of treatment) in a group when compared to a similar group without access to that intervention, but without using a random allocation process. It is a flexible way to carry out research in the real world, where the random allocation of participants (as in randomised controlled trials) in a study proves difficult for one reason or another.

KEY POINTS

- Participants are not randomly allocated to groups in quasi-experimental designs
- Interpretation of the results of quasi-experimental studies should be done with caution, due to threats to internal and external validity
- Quasi-experiments are useful in the real world where the random allocation of subjects to a control group is not feasible due to ethical or other justifiable reasons
- Careful planning of a quasi-experimental study can minimise the risk of other confounding factors (other than the intervention) influencing the outcome

DISCUSSION

The main purpose of any research is to find answers to difficult questions and better solutions for problems affecting our lives. In an ideal world, this can be achieved by carrying out proper experiments comparing the effects of a treatment or intervention in two or more identical groups. Participants should be randomly allocated to treatment and control groups and assessed, without bias, using reliable and valid measures. Unfortunately, this is not always possible.

Evaluating the impact of an independent variable such as smoking or drinking on health will cause concern to participants if they are randomly allocated to the experimental group with an expectation that they smoke or drink as part of the study. Similarly, to assess differences in people of different ethnic or religious backgrounds (subject variables that you can't change), random allocation becomes irrelevant.

There are other circumstances too, such as when an intervention (to be evaluated by research) has already been introduced within the population as a part of health policy or where randomly allocating participants (patients) to a non-treatment (control) group is likely to deteriorate their condition and so is completely unjustifiable for ethical reasons. Here, planning research based on 'proper' experimental design becomes unacceptable. Quasi-experimental design studies are therefore necessary in these and many other circumstances in healthcare.

Quasi-experimental design types

Single group studies

These are sometimes carried out as convenient pilot studies, forming pre-experimental designs. The value of findings in such studies is questionable. Examples of single group studies are as follows.

- **Single group post-test study** – A single post-intervention assessment forms the basis of judging the efficacy of treatment. An example of this would be making an assumption about the effectiveness of cognitive behavioural therapy (CBT) for depression based on the depression score recorded in a group of depressed patients in a surgery after receiving a course of CBT. As the researcher has no idea of the patients' depression scores prior to commencing CBT, however, a single post-test assessment would be meaningless for all practical purposes.
- **Single group pre- and post-test study** – In the above example, the group's baseline (pre-treatment) depression score would be assessed and any decline in the post-CBT depression score would form the basis of a judgement of the effectiveness of the treatment. Conclusions based on such studies have major pitfalls. As there is only one reference baseline and one outcome measure, it can't be deduced whether or not these are reliable results and factors other than CBT are influencing the results of the study.

Time series

In this design, a series of observations of the experimental group are carried out pre- and post-intervention (treatment). Time series, by its nature, is a longitudinal study where repeated observations (up to 50 or more) are made. These observations help in finding if there is a definite trend before and after the intervention. This kind of design is often used in social and public health research.

When the intervention is stopped and started during the time series observations, the design is called 'interrupted time series'. If the trend of observations is in the same direction after each episode of intervention and vice versa, this gives stronger evidence of the effectiveness of the intervention. For example, in one study using interrupted time series design, Fuller et al. (2012) found that two London Underground train strikes led to an increase in the use of bikes.

Two (non-equivalent control) groups study design

This design attempts to compare two groups, one with an intervention (experimental) and one without (control). Participants in these groups are not randomly assigned. This gives rise to non-equivalent groups. An example might be that of examining the effect of a health education programme on obesity in male A-level students in a state school compared to male A-level students in a neighbouring private school. Differences in their social backgrounds or school environments could be important confounding factors influencing the outcome of this study.

Case-control design

The strategy most commonly used to minimise the differences between two comparison groups in quasi-experimental studies is that of researchers matching participants based on one or more variables in their control group. In the above example, for instance, the boys from private schools taken for the study could be matched for their social class.

The difference between this type of design and the experimental design is that here the control group as a whole is predetermined, whereas in the experimental design, participants are matched and then randomly allocated to the experimental and control group.

Regression discontinuity design

In this design, two groups are divided by a cut-off point value of a certain variable based on arbitrary criteria. Their pre-test and post-test measures are displayed on either side of the cut-off point. The impact of the programme is measured by the shift in post-test measures to above a projected continuous line across the two groups. The scattered observations are entered along a projected line (regression) and the continuity of the projected line will be shifted (discontinuity) if the intervention has any effect.

This kind of design is often used to evaluate the impact of a programme targeted at a needy population. In that way, one group with participants below a certain value are used as the intervention group and the control group contains participants who are above the certain value. For example, in a special needs school, all subjects with an IQ below 80 could form one group that needs a special education package (intervention group) and the rest with an IQ over 80 could be included in a control group. Their scholastic performance could then be measured after the intervention package and, if they showed more improvement than expected, the result would look like that shown in Figure 28.1.

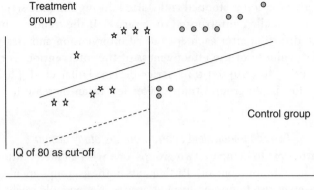

Figure 28.1 Scholastic performance after an intervention programme, showing use of regression discontinuity design

Ludwig and Miller (2007) used this design to evaluate the impact of the Head Start programme on children's lives in the poorest counties in the USA. Shadish et al. (2011) found that the results of regression discontinuity design studies can be as robust as those produced by experimental designs.

Stepped-wedge design

Here, clusters of participants are assigned to a treatment group in a staggered fashion at random intervals. They are therefore considered a control group until they enter into the treatment phase. Each cluster eventually receives the intervention. The stepped-wedge design is therefore a cluster-randomised type of crossover design (Handley et al., 2011).

This kind of design is useful in real-world research where intervention programmes are introduced in stages. The waiting times for the groups of individuals to receive the intervention are taken as the control. Figure 28.2 give an example of a stepped-wedge design, the shaded cells representing an intervention period, the blank cells a control period and the bottom row (1–6) the data collection points.

Correlational design

Correlational studies indicate strong associations between variables and the event under investigation. A causal relationship is nothing more than a presumption. For example, if a study finds that children who watch violent video games also show increased evidence of aggressive behaviour, this could mean that watching violent video games leads to aggressive behaviour. This is rather a premature conclusion, however, as there may be other factors responsible for their behaviour.

Correlational studies are a useful addition to research designs used in the real world for longitudinal, naturalistic studies. The proposed causal links based on these studies can be further examined by means of experimental studies.

Participants/
clusters

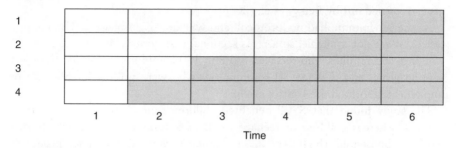

Figure 28.2 Example of a stepped-wedge design

Limitations of quasi-experimental design

Campbell and Stanley (1963), while emphasising the value of quasi-experimental studies, also highlight some drawbacks. A number of factors may affect the change in the variable under study other than the intervention, thus making the results questionable. These are considered threats to internal validity and could be one or more of the following.

- **Historical** – Unexpected events that occurred during the study period influencing the outcome, such as the outbreak of an illness affecting one group of participants. The single group design is even more vulnerable to this threat.
- **Maturation** – A natural change occurring in participants that has a positive or negative effect on outcomes, such as the effect of getting old on physical ability.
- **Selection** – Two groups are unequal so that other confounding variables determine the outcome more than the intervention being researched.
- **Statistical regression** – Where groups have participants with extreme scores at the start of the study, they will have a tendency to move towards the mean as the study progresses, thus influencing the outcome.
- **Tests and bias** – If participants learn how to respond to the measurement scales used before or during the study, they may invalidate the results. In some instances, they may respond positively to please the researcher.

Certain factors in quasi-experiments may lead to study results that can't be applied to a wider population. These are therefore considered threats to external validity. This kind of threat arises when the participant group is not representative of the population the study findings are to be applied to or when the study environment influences the results so much that they can't be applied in a real-world situation.

CASE STUDY

The Sure Start Local Programme (SSLP) was introduced by the UK government to improve the health and well-being of young children in deprived communities in England in 1999. As the government ruled out an experimental study to evaluate the effectiveness of the programme, a quasi-experimental design was planned instead, carried out by Belsky et al. (2006).

As the programme had no 'protocol' and was already in place, systematic pre-test data was not available, so a cross-sectional case control design was planned. Children and families who received SSLP in 150 communities formed the intervention group and those in 50 communities who were waiting for SSLP to be implemented formed the control group.

The study found that SSLP benefited children from relatively less deprived families, whereas children of teenage mothers, lone parents or coming from a workless household (high-deprivation families) were, if anything, negatively affected by SSLP. The health team-led SSLP had a more positive effect than the program led by local authorities or other agencies.

This case study highlights the difficulty of planning an experimental study for such programmes and the need for quasi-experimental studies for health or other programmes introduced without a sound evidence base. The studies can be improved by collecting pre-test data in both groups, making the programme (intervention) more standardised with a defined protocol, extending the study so that the control group turns into the intervention group (stepped-wedge design) in order to evaluate the long-term effect of the intervention, as well as enhance internal and external validity.

CONCLUSION

Quasi-experimental design is necessary in real-world research. Studies, if properly planned, can minimise the threats to internal and external validity.

FURTHER READING

Cook, T.D. and Campbell, D.T. (1979) *Quasi-experimentation: Design and analysis issues for field settings*. Boston, MA: Houghton Mifflin.

REFERENCES

Belsky, J., Melhuish, E., Barnes, J., Leyland A.H. and Romaniuk, H. (2006) 'Effects of Sure Start Local Programmes on children and families: Early findings from a quasi-experimental, cross-sectional study', *British Medical Journal*, 332 (7556): 1476–8.

Campbell, D.T. and Stanley, J.C. (1963) *Experimental and Quasi-experimental Designs for Research*. Chicago, IL: Rand McNally.

Fuller, D., Sahlqvist, S., Cummins, S. and Ogilvie, D. (2012) 'The impact of public transportation strikes on use of a bicycle share programme in London: Interrupted time series design', *Preventive Medicine*, 54 (1): 74–6.

Handley, M.A., Schillinger, D. and Shiboski, S. (2011) 'Quasi-experimental designs in practice-based research settings: Design and implementation considerations', *Journal of the American Board of Family Medicine*, 24 (5): 589–96.

Ludwig, J. and Miller, D.L. (2007) 'Does Head Start improve children's life changes?: Evidence from a regression discontinuity design', *The Quarterly Journal of Economics*, 122 (1): 159–208.

Shadish, W.R., Galindo, R., Wong, V.C., Steiner, P.M. and Cook T.D. (2011) 'A randomized experiment comparing random and cutoff-based assignment', *Psychological Methods*, 16 (2): 179–91.

29 Survey Research

Simon Alford

DEFINITION

Can you measure it? Can you express it in figures? Can you make a model of it? If not, your theory is apt to be based more upon imagination than upon knowledge.

(Lord Kelvin, cited in Lacombe, 2005: 1)

A 'survey' is a system employed to collect information to describe, compare or explain knowledge, attitudes and behaviours (Fink, 1995). In doing so, a survey investigates an area of interest, gathering a sample of data that will allow a comprehensive view that is representative of the population being studied.

KEY POINTS

- Surveys can be useful to assess and understand attitudes, behaviours or risk factors of a population or subsample in relation to health. Responses can be quantified in order to help support service development
- There is a range of survey methodologies available and it is important that the advantages and disadvantages of each method are weighed up to ensure the most appropriate method is selected
- The design of a survey instrument itself is of fundamental importance. It is essential to keep things simple and at an appropriate level to ensure respondents can answer each question to allow meaningful conclusions to be drawn
- Surveys are typically undertaken with a sample of the population of interest in order to draw conclusions that can be applied to the wider population

29 survey research

153

- Surveys are notorious for mixed response rates. A range of techniques can be incorporated to help encourage responses, while piloting is essential to help ensure reliable measurements are obtained

DISCUSSION

Surveys and their application

The number of surveys conducted each year is huge, with studies undertaken to assess opinions on myriad topics. Often they are undertaken to gauge public opinion or gain insights into consumers' preferences and to support organisational management, policy development and service provision.

Survey methodology is commonly used in research and can help to provide information on a range of measurements, but there are potential stumbling blocks that need to be overcome in order to produce good-quality research. A sound research design makes a research question researchable, allows the study to produce specific answers to specific questions and, ultimately, makes it possible to draw valid conclusions from the data collected. Trying to answer too many things can result in none of the questions being fully explored (Coughlan et al., 2009).

Survey delivery methods

There are three main ways in which surveys are carried out:

- interviews, whether face to face or by telephone
- observation
- questionnaires – either posted to people or online.

While these three methods all have the same aim of eliciting information, there are advantages and disadvantages with each method.

Interviews can be effective at engaging participants/respondents and can be conducted either face to face or by telephone. Telephone interviews are becoming more commonplace and have been demonstrated to provide comparable data to those from face-to-face interviews (Sturges and Hanrahan, 2004).

Interviews for survey purposes traditionally rely on a structured approach to ensure standardisation, especially when multiple researchers are conducting the interviews. While the interviewers can help ensure participants fully understand the questions, they can be time-consuming and costly.

Observations are a less common form of survey research, but, for example, there are traffic censuses and investigations into pedestrian flows which are commonly used when looking to establish venues for new shops, identifying the potential footfall (Aldridge and Levine, 2001). As with interviews, conducting observational research can involve a significant time element.

Questionnaires are the most commonly used survey method and can take a range of formats, including postal, self-administered and group-administered.

Since the late 1990s, however, the development of technology and the ever-growing popularity of the Internet and social media has seen a rise in the number of electronic surveys/questionnaires being conducted (Van Gelder et al., 2010).

Initially, electronic questionnaires were either embedded within or attached to e-mail notifications that allowed participants to also respond via e-mail. The past decade, however, has seen a significant rise in the popularity of surveys conducted via websites (surveymonkey, smart-survey and so on). Despite the use of questionnaires being common practice, each method of administrating them has a number of advantages and disadvantages, as examined below.

Postal questionnaires have the potential to reach people over a wide area, but can appear impersonal and have serious cost implications, especially with large-scale surveys. Further issues with postal surveys include the challenge of low response rates, especially among certain populations. Issues around poor literacy/visual impairment, the inability of respondents to ask questions and incomplete questionnaires can also be problematic.

Self-administered questionnaires are a low-cost option, but it is unlikely that a researcher will be able to reach people over a wide area. One advantage is that they allow respondents to ask questions, which can support good completion rates.

Group-administered questionnaires have benefits in relation to cost and completion rates for large assembled groups. It is difficult, however, to reach people over a wide area and more difficult to answer individuals' questions to ensure completion than when dealing with respondents individually. Furthermore, respondents in a group situation can talk to each other while completing the questionnaire, which can influence the outcomes.

E-mail questionnaires also have the potential to reduce costs, be easily administered and allow access to a large (worldwide) population. They also have the potential to elicit higher-quality responses at a faster rate than postal or self-administered questionnaires. A lack of computer literacy and anonymity could affect levels of engagement, however, while coverage, sampling errors and non-deliverability may prevent a representative sample from being achieved (Fan and Yan, 2010).

Website questionnaires are a significant further development of the e-mail questionnaire. In addition to the potential to reduce costs, ease the amount of administration required and provide access to a large population, website questionnaires reduce the need for manual data entry associated with paper-based surveys (Fan and Yan, 2010). They also allow respondents to be directed by means of relevant questions based on their responses and targeted reminders to be sent to non-respondents.

The disadvantages of e-mail questionnaires identified above are true of website questionnaires, too, while issues concerning computer safety and security have become more prevalent. Such challenges can result in a sample being non-representative, which then limits the ability to infer the applicability of any results to a wider population.

Survey design

In order to conduct a survey, an appropriate measurement tool is required. It is essential to have a well-designed survey tool if the right information is going to be obtained to draw meaningful conclusions.

There are two main types of survey. First, there are 'descriptive surveys', such as opinion polls and censuses, which are used for prediction purposes and set out to count (for example, age, sex, ethnicity, income) and find facts by sampling an entire population or a representative sample.

Second, there are 'analytical surveys', which infer relationships between variables and use questions to examine the 'why' in order to identify differences between or within groups.

When designing surveys, most questions are either 'open' or 'closed'. Closed questions provide a fixed set of responses to choose from (such as Likert scales or simply 'Yes' and 'No' options), which are easy to analyse quantitatively. A disadvantage of closed questions, however, is that they can be too simplistic, inflexible and lack a sense of depth (Bryman, 2012). Open questions can gain more insight by eliciting more expressive responses, but can take longer to answer, longer to code and, subsequently, longer to analyse.

When using a questionnaire, it is important that the focus and content of the questions is correct and the sequence they are put into does not influence subsequent questions. The wording of the questions should also be suitable for its audience. This is especially important when working with children or groups of people who have low levels of literacy. It should also be remembered that a number of survey tools have already been produced and validated and these can often be used with the author's permission, which can save time and be more reliable than constructing your own. This option is not appropriate for all research, however, especially when examining relatively new and novel topics or when looking to develop existing research.

Populations and sampling

When undertaking a survey, it is necessary to define the 'population', which is all the individuals who fall into the category of interest relating to the research question. Unless we are trying to gain the views of the nation, as with the national census traditionally conducted once every ten years, a 'sample' of that population will need to be found. To allow conclusions to be drawn that can be applied to a wider population, the sample will need to be a 'representative sample' – that is, those in this group have similar characteristics to the whole of that population. If the sample is to be truly representative, it implies that every member of that population has an equal chance of being asked to participate (Oppenheim, 1992).

Where possible, the sample should be as large as possible to help with the precision of the survey, although factors including the availability of postal addresses, e-mail addresses, telephone numbers, time and cost can have serious implications for the size of a sample. A simple technique is to place each individual's name in a hat and draw out names randomly. While this technique is acceptable for small-scale studies, it is not practical for larger surveys. Traditionally, larger samples have been drawn from lists, such as telephone directories. As populations are more transient than they used to be and mobile phone usage has increased, resulting in fewer people being listed in directories, the recruitment and retention of participants has become more and more challenging (Blumberg and Luke, 2011).

In an ideal scenario, sample populations would be truly representative, which would reduce the levels of bias within the results. For many small-scale or student research projects, however, the samples are often non-representative and convenience tends to play a role in selection. In general, recruiting subjects to take part in such studies has become more problematic, with strategies such as systematic knocking on doors, advertising for volunteers and school- or service-based recruitment having their own limitations, including response rates (Morton et al., 2006).

Data collection

Before diving into collecting data, it is important to undertake some pilot work, trialling the survey with a small number of people. Ideally, piloting should involve people from the desired population to ensure that the planned procedures are workable and appropriate, the measurement tool is assessing what it is intended to measure and it is reliable. Without pilot work there is the possibility that time, money and effort could be wasted, carrying out a study that has no chance of being successful. This is also in itself unethical.

It is important to consider the timeframe for responses using the various techniques. As Hoonakker and Carayon (2009) suggest, the speed of response for e-mail (7.7 days) and web-based surveys (6.7 days) are considerably quicker than for postal surveys (16.1 days). Despite the variations in response times, website surveys have been found to have similar response rates to postal surveys – 52 v 51 per cent, compared to 32 per cent for e-mail surveys.

There are various techniques that can be used to try and minimise the numbers of people who don't respond. These include:

- giving advance warning
- clear explanation letters
- confidentiality
- survey design
- length of questionnaire
- incentives (prize draw entry)
- reminders and return envelopes.

It should also be acknowledged that response rates can be dependent on the topic of the survey and the population selected.

CASE STUDY

The Health Survey for England (HSE) was first introduced in 1991 and has been conducted annually to provide regular information on various aspects of the nation's health. A random sample of approximately 30,000 addresses in England are selected based on 720 postcode sectors. The survey combines questionnaire-based answers, interviews and physical measurements, which include the analysis of blood samples.

The HSE aims to provide a representative sample of the population in England who have specified health conditions and estimate the prevalence of certain risk factors as well as combinations of risk factors associated with these conditions.

CONCLUSION

This chapter has described a range of research strategies that can be employed when undertaking survey work and the associated issues that can have implications for the timescale and cost implications of a research project. The areas covered give a foundation for understanding when and how a survey may be beneficial and the need to engage and capture the target audience. It should also be remembered that surveys can be incorporated within other research strategies.

FURTHER READING

Andres, L. (2012) *Designing and Doing Survey Research*. London: Sage.
Sue, V.M. and Ritter, L.A. (2007) *Conducting Online Surveys*. London: Sage.

REFERENCES

Aldridge, A. and Levine, K. (2001) *Surveying the Social World: Principles and practice in survey research*. Buckingham: Open University Press.
Blumberg, S.J. and Luke, J.V. (2011) 'Wireless substitution: Estimates from the National Health Interview Survey, January–June 2011'. Hyattsville, MD: Centers for Disease Control and Prevention (available online at: www.cdc.gov/nchs/nhis/releases.htm#wireless).
Bryman, A. (2012) *Social Research Methods*. Oxford: Oxford University Press.
Coughlan, M., Cronin, P. and Ryan, F. (2009) 'Survey research: Process and limitations', *International Journal of Therapy and Rehabilitation*, 16: 9–15.
Fan, W. and Yan, Z. (2010) 'Factors affecting response rates of the web survey: A systematic review', *Computers in Human Behavior*, 26: 132–9.
Fink, A. (1995) *How to Analyze Survey Data*. Thousand Oaks, CA: Sage.
Hoonakker, P. and Carayon, P. (2009) 'Questionnaire survey nonresponse: A comparison of postal mail and internet surveys', *International Journal of Human–Computer Interaction*, 25: 348–73.
Lacombe, R. (2005) *Adhesion Measurement Methods: Theory and practice*. Florida, CA: CRC Press.
Morton, L.M., Cahill, J. and Hartge, P. (2006) 'Reporting participation in epidemiologic studies: A survey of practice', *American Journal of Epidemiology*, 163: 197–203.
Oppenheim, A.N. (1992) *Questionnaire Design, Interviewing and Attitude Measurement*. London: Continuum.
Sturges, J. and Hanrahan, K. (2004) 'Comparing telephone and face-to-face qualitative interviewing: A research note', *Qualitative Research*, 4: 107–18.
Van Gelder, M., Bretveld, R. and Roeleveld, N. (2010) 'Web-based questionnaires: The future in epidemiology?', *American Journal of Epidemiology*, 72: 1292–8.

30 Hypotheses

Stephen Fallows

DEFINITION

An 'hypothesis' (plural hypotheses) is a testable statement that describes a likely relationship between an independent and one or more dependent variables. It is the testing of the hypothesis that provides the basis of much quantitative research. An hypothesis can be presented in either the null or alternative form, as explained below.

KEY POINTS

- An hypothesis is a tentative proposition, not established theory
- It must be capable of being tested

DISCUSSION

Much quantitative research begins with the development of an hypothesis or hypotheses based on past observations and a hunch that relationships exist between variables. Such relationships are of a limited range of general forms:

- a measurable change to variable A will lead to a measurable change in variable B
- different types of variable C will be associated with different (usually measurable or at least observable) characteristics regarding variable D.

The aim of the research is to challenge the hypothesis to determine whether or not evidence supports the statement.

Hypothesis development (including case studies)

Formulating an hypothesis can often prove to be quite difficult. It is useful to illustrate this with a few examples given as case studies.

Case study 1

A student making a first attempt at developing an hypothesis might suggest, for example, 'A change in habitual daily exercise will lead to a change in heart rate'. This statement takes us part way to having an hypothesis, but a number of points need to be addressed.

- What sort of change in exercise level is envisaged? What degree of intensity? What period of time?
- How long will the study continue?
- Who is doing the exercise?
- When is heart rate to be measured? At rest or after an exercise session?
- What is the expected direction of change?

The student may revise the hypothesis to 'Adoption of 30 minutes brisk walking daily for 6 weeks will lower the resting heart rate for elderly men who have recently experienced a myocardial infarction'. Here, there is a much clearer indication of the specific circumstances of the proposed study. Of course, some questions still remain (for example, about how 'elderly' is defined and what exactly is meant by 'recently experienced' and if the patients' post-MI treatment regime is relevant), but the hypothesis is testable. There is a clear experimental intervention (addition of the walk to the daily habits – that is, is there a walk or not) and a clearly defined outcome measure.

Case study 2

A second student offers the idea that 'Relaxation classes have an impact on level of stress and lead to improved happiness'. Again, there is a need to unpick the initial proposition to yield true hypotheses.

The first thing to note is that, although there is a single independent variable – attendance at the relaxation classes – there are two dependent variables (measurable outcomes) stress level and happiness. Having two dependent variables is problematic as attendance at the classes may have an influence on stress levels, but no impact on happiness (or vice versa). The student should split the idea to yield two separate hypotheses:

- attendance at relaxation classes has an impact on stress levels
- attendance at relaxation classes has an impact on happiness.

Each of these hypotheses can now be tested independently and there is the possibility it is a change in stress level that is impacting happiness quite separately from the relaxation classes.

As with Case study 1, the hypotheses can be refined further by addition of, for example, details about the participants and the nature and number of classes. The student could also be more specific about the manner in which stress and happiness are to be defined.

Case study 3

A third student indicates an interest in comparing boys' and girls' performances in a test designed to assess knowledge of nutrition. The student thinks that girls will be more knowledgeable than boys, but has no justification for this hunch.

While an hypothesis can be constructed – 'Girls will score more highly than boys in a nutrition knowledge test' – it may be more appropriate at this exploratory stage to base the study on a question, such as, 'Which have the highest scores in a nutrition knowledge test, boys or girls?'

Case study 4

For some quantitative studies, the nature of the work and data to be collected do not easily lend themselves to the use of hypotheses. A study that simply seeks to determine the height and weight of a defined group of teenagers is much better presented as a question. If, however, the study then sought to compare the heights and weights with published standards, then hypotheses would become appropriate.

Presentation of hypotheses

All of the examples given above are presented in the 'experimental' or 'alternative' format, but it is usual, when moving on to test hypotheses statistically, to use the 'null' format. Essentially, this revises the form of the hypothesis statement so that it says there is no relationship or no difference. The hypotheses in our examples above would then read as follows.

- The addition of exercise will have no impact on resting heart rate.
- Attendance at relaxation classes has no impact on level of stress.
- There will be no difference between boys' and girls' scores in a nutrition knowledge test.
- Heights (or weights) of the measured teenagers will be no different those predicted by looking at published norms.

Appropriate statistical analysis aims to determine whether the available evidence allows for the hypothesis to be supported or rejected. Such support or rejection is presented with an indication of the likelihood that evidence is stronger than would be expected by chance (see Chapter 33, Statistics: Inferential).

In some documents, the null hypothesis is designated H0, with the experimental or alternative designated H1.

In the example hypotheses given above, there is a clear indication of the direction of the expected change or difference – a decrease in the expected resting heart rate, a decrease in stress level, an increase in happiness and girls scoring higher than boys. Such hypotheses are referred to as 'one-tailed'. Where there is no prediction of direction, then the term 'two-tailed' is used.

Rejection of the hypothesis

In most instances, hypotheses are accepted or rejected on the basis of the outcomes of appropriate statistical analysis. If the analysis leads to rejection of the null hypothesis (there is no relationship between variable A and variable B), then the evidence is suggestive of the predicted relationship holding true. It should not therefore be taken that there is a *proof* of the relationship – merely, the current state of our knowledge continues to support the hypothesis.

There are some hypotheses for which the overwhelming amount of recorded evidence provides support. Examples include such simple and seemingly definitive statements as:

- when an object is dropped it will fall
- all swans are white.

The first of these statements remained 'true' – that is, the hypothesis was supported – until the start of the era of travel into space. From that time onwards, the hypothesis needed to be changed as an object dropped *in zero gravity* does *not* fall. This is a further example of the need for hypotheses to be stated with due reference to the circumstances of the observation. In this instance, the hypothesis continues to be supported in conditions where there is gravity (such as on Earth), but not in the very different conditions of zero gravity in space.

The second statement would have been supported by Europeans for millennia – this was what they would have observed. When black swans were reported in Australia, however, the position was immediately found to be false. This illustrates very clearly how a single (previously, seemingly impossible) observation can, on occasion, lead to the rejection of even long-established positions.

It is also important to note the difference between two quite different concepts:

- no evidence of black swans
- evidence of no black swans.

Statements in the former format may be finally verifiable as false (as when the black swans were found in Australia). The second statement is not so simple to resolve.

The existence of black swans can be related to new circumstances surrounding observations – in this case, the observations were on a different continent.

The above illustrates how an hypothesis is only valid in the contexts of its place and circumstances. All hypotheses stand or fall on the basis of the current state of our knowledge and circumstances. It is common for long-supported hypotheses to fall away as research moves on and this is especially so as new measurement techniques provide new means of data collection.

Hypotheses, theories and laws

'Hypotheses' can be described as 'hunches' or 'educated guesses' (I prefer the latter). Each hypothesis is constructed by researchers on the basis of consideration of past formal knowledge (drawn from published research) and personal experience, stirred together with individual opinion on how this can be interpreted and developed into new studies.

'Theories' come later in the process. They draw on a number of hypotheses in an area of research and summarise the outcomes to build a more general concept.

The issue of how diet might impact cardiovascular health provides a useful case example. The following is a very much abbreviated summary of the progression of ideas on this topic.

- Epidemiological theorists suggested hypotheses about the relationship between national statistics on dietary patterns and national data on morbidity and mortality from cardiovascular disease.
- Further hypotheses were developed linking:
  - o diet constituents with plasma levels of lipids
  - o lipid levels with development of pathological conditions, such as atherosclerosis
  - o pathological measurements with overt clinical conditions (angina, myocardial infarction and so on).
- Clinical trials tested hypotheses that related to the modification of diets with a view to recording the clinical outcomes for patients.
- Clinicians and others reviewed the evidence from the many sources and developed the advice that is promulgated by health bodies worldwide.

In the above sequence, researchers addressed a series of individual hypotheses and each built on previous work. The current theory with respect to the role of lipids is based on a rather strong set of hypotheses that are supported by the available evidence. We still need to remember, however, that new evidence my cause the rejection of one or more of the currently supported fundamental hypotheses and result in a cascade of new thinking.

While 'theories' remain open to challenge, it is common for those with sceptical views to refer to (even long established) theories using the term 'hypothesis'. So, the cardiovascular scenario outlined above is commonly referred to as the 'fats hypothesis' by those who seek to suggest alternative hypotheses.

'Laws' are the step beyond theories, bringing us as close to certainty (facts) as we are able to be. This is where every element of research evidence confirms the established position. Infectious disease, for example, provides many strong examples of exposure to a specified infectious agent leading to the named condition. Regarding the cardiovascular example above, however, we are not yet in the position of agreeing definitive laws.

CONCLUSION

The testing of one hypothesis or more is a key feature of most quantitative research. Hypotheses are accepted (for the present time) or rejected on the basis of the analysis of appropriate data. Further research may overturn previously accepted hypotheses. In time, collections of hypotheses build to yield theories and, if unchallenged over time, theories may become laws.

FURTHER READING

Taleb, N.N. (2007) *The Black Swan: The impact of the highly improbable.* London: Penguin.

31 Measurement Instruments

Andrew E.P. Mitchell

DEFINITION

'Measurement instruments' in research are about allocating numbers to quantify something that is of interest to practitioners.

In healthcare research, it is important to measure some things because they are about some aspect or characteristic of the patients' future well-being or ill health. The characteristics may be directly observable, such as height and weight, but are more likely to be less available to direct observation because of their complexity. In these cases, the measurement instruments are used to infer or represent a closely related characteristic in the patient that is of potential interest.

The very characteristics that can be potentially the most informative to practitioners are often completely unavailable to direct observation, and include those involved with anxiety, depression and related aspects, such as people's thoughts or attitudes that affect well-being (Beck, 2011). These so-called 'abstract' concepts do not lend themselves easily to measurement, but useful standard measurement techniques are available to help practitioners to quantify characteristics of interest or aid in the development of such instruments.

For many such characteristics, healthcare professionals tend to rely on either observational or self-reports that measure the relative amount of the characteristic and enable some form of comparison to be made between them and others with this characteristic. The allocation of numerical scores to the characteristic is central to this process.

The challenge for practitioners in all this is that of constructing valid measurement instruments for characteristics that cannot be measured directly. Such characteristics often include unhelpful attitudes patients hold towards certain health behaviours or the ways in which individuals think about events in their everyday lives, ways that can contribute to anxiety or depressive states (Beck, 2011).

KEY POINTS

- Measurement instruments enable the quantification of characteristics of interest to researchers
- There are several methods of measuring characteristics, including scaling techniques

- Any measurement instrument must be valid and reliable
- Measurement instruments are important in healthcare research as they enable the measurement of attributes that are difficult to observe directly, such as cognitive and affective characteristics

DISCUSSION

Measurement techniques and scaling

There are several ways to measure attitudes or the ways in which people think about things, but the most popular are the self-reporting (individuals rating themselves) or observer reporting (practitioners rating the individuals) methods – both involve some form of scaling technique.

Scaling techniques can involve unipolar or bipolar points, which can be numbered or anchored with clear descriptions or degrees of the characteristics being investigated. The most popular are the Likert and semantic differential scales.

Likert scales
Dr Rensis Likert (1932) devised what has become popularly known as the Likert scale. It is designed to provide a valid or accurate measure of individuals' attitudes towards an object or concept. It requires respondents to indicate a degree of agreement or disagreement with each of a series of statements related to the attitude or concept being measured. For example:

Strongly agree   Agree   Unsure   Disagree   Strongly disagree

To analyse a Likert scale, each response category is assigned a numerical value. The example above could be assigned values such as Strongly agree = +2, through to Strongly disagree = –2. Each individual Likert scale can be analysed on an item-by-item basis or a number of individual Likert scales on the same topic could be summed to form a single score for that topic as a whole.

Semantic differential scale
Charles Osgood et al.'s (1957) semantic differential scale was designed to measure the connotative meaning of concepts. The instrument consists of a number of bipolar adjectives, such as good/bad, pleasant/unpleasant, fair/unfair and so on. As with the Likert scale, there is a continuum, but here the endpoints are the bipolar opposites of each other and the midpoint is the neutral position:

Good   1   2   3   4   5   6   7   Bad

Unlike the Likert scale, the semantic differential scale, by providing these bipolar pairs of words, asks respondents to indicate on a continuum a particular aspect of their attitudes towards the topic being investigated.

Using the results of scales

The scaling techniques allow an estimate to be made of the characteristic of interest, but practitioners must be aware of measurement reliability issues.

The sum score for these techniques is normally made up of a true score, accurate measure of the characteristic and an error score, representing issues that might compromise accurate measuring of the characteristic of interest. These issues must be recognised and addressed by researchers.

Psychological measurement: attitudinal scaling

The measurement of attitudes in healthcare is important when looking at health behaviours or changing unhelpful attitudes towards interventions designed to bring about health benefits.

The majority of attitudes that people hold towards certain health behaviours are not always as transparent as we might first imagine. For example, people might *say* they want to help alleviate their depressed mood by engaging in certain helpful activities – sometimes called 'behavioural activation' – but when they are about to engage in the behaviour, they feel unable to do so. Therefore, there is a need for measurement instruments that assess the three components of an attitude – that is, the affective, behavioural and cognitive components of the ABC model (Rosenberg and Hovland, 1960).

The 'affective component' can be described as the feelings that the person has about the new behaviour. The 'behavioural component' is the actions or behaviours that the person takes to begin the new activity. The 'cognitive component' is the thoughts or images that the person has towards the action. The ABC model implies that the cognitive component will be highly correlated with the behavioural and affective components.

There are some caveats to the idea that attitudes could possibly be predictive of how a person feels or suggest what the person is thinking or what behaviour is likely to result from holding such attitudes. It is likely that general attitudes will only allow for general predictions as to how a person is likely to behave because other variables, such as the current situation, may limit demonstration of the attitude–behaviour link in the everyday context. A congregation of similar beliefs, however, is likely to energise or overcome situational factors and is more predictive of resultant behaviours and feelings than just one (Ajzen and Fishbein, 1977).

Key principles

The allocation of numerical scores to the characteristic of interest is the first stage, but some scaling of the characteristic is an essential prerequisite.

The grouping of properties into categories, such as healthy eaters and unhealthy eaters, is helpful and this is called 'nominal scaling'. Such scaling, though helpful, is limited, due to the lack of knowledge about how the properties are to be ordered along a defined measurement scale.

It is sometimes possible to rank the characteristic according to information about its magnitude and this is called 'ordinal scaling'. It is this type of scaling that is the main focus of the techniques discussed so far in this chapter.

The next level of scaling, which is not always achievable in attitudinal scales, but is sometimes possible, says something about the ranking order and the size of the magnitude between each point within the scale. This is called 'interval scaling'.

Whether the scaling used is classified as ordinal or interval scaling is important when thinking about and applying the most appropriate statistical tests (Greene and D'Oliveira, 2006).

Another key principle is checking that the intended scale is valid and reliable. Scaling techniques do not necessarily result in valid measurement instruments, so researchers need to check that the instrument they are using is measuring what it purports to measure. The standard procedure is to select or develop a series of question items that are known to represent the characteristic that is of interest. This process is sometimes known as 'operationalisation' of the characteristic and involves recourse to the available literature for definitions of the variable being investigated. Operationalisation is the process of making the concept more precise by linking it to one or more standard indicators or agreed on definitions. The reliability of the measure is its ability to consistently report similar results each time it is used under the same conditions. The scaling of the characteristic and operationalisation of concepts are important when designing an appropriate measurement instrument that is both valid and reliable.

The Likert and semantic differential scales often involve a number of direct and sometimes searching questions, which may lead to social desirability effects and, to a lesser extent, response sets. If the purpose of the measurement instrument is obvious to respondents, depending on the focus of the attitudinal scale, they may want to confirm or answer in a socially desirable manner rather than give their true views on the topic. 'Response sets' are when respondents consistently agree or disagree without focusing on the individual questions.

The giving of socially desirable responses can be minimised by making the intention of the scale less obvious by including items not related to the attitude that is the focus of the question or study. Other techniques include assuring respondents anonymity and confidentiality regarding their responses.

The issue of response set can be problematic in poorly designed scales. This can be largely overcome, however, by wording items randomly to represent counterbalance responses in unfavourable or favourable directions. This encourages respondents to read each item carefully to ascertain the attitudinal direction.

CASE STUDY

The use of measurement instruments in healthcare research comes into its own when investigating concepts that cannot be measured directly, such as the cognitive and affective characteristics. Mitchell (2012) designed a series of studies to extend knowledge of the cognitive and affective characteristics involved in memory retrieval.

The studies observed the effect that negative mood has on the recall of memories by using a measurement instrument to quantify cognitive and affective aspects. A modified version of the autobiographical memory test (AMT) (Williams and

Broadbent, 1986) was used. This test has been widely used to assess autobiographical content and has been found to have a good level of reliability (Williams et al., 2007).

The technique involves a participant being supplied with cue words and, after each, being asked to recall a memory associated with that word. Mitchell (2012) examined participants' memories in this way by asking them to rate each cued memory recalled in the negative mood state on a Likert scale, similar in design to the scaling techniques discussed above. The participants rated their cued memories using endorsements such as emotionality, personal importance and expectancy.

Mitchell identified the dominant characteristics in autobiographical memory and constructed a number of single-item questions to assess the dimensions of interest. It is also possible to use item pools, similar questions related to the target characteristic or a single item that corresponds to the variable of interest to do this. One of the single-item questions asked was, 'Was the event expected?', which was mapped with a similar question on the impact of future events scale (IFES) (Deeprose and Holmes, 2010), a validated measure, to assess the attribute of future predictability.

The participants rated the single items and endorsed the statements on a seven-point Likert scale. The endorsements were observed pre- and post-negative mood, the mood having been induced and observed against four components of negative mood, as measured by the University of Wales Institute of Science and Technology's mood adjective checklist (UWIST-MACL) (Matthews et al., 1990). Such mapping can be helpful in operationalising the characteristics of interest and could possibly strengthen the validity of the content of a study.

The results of such mood state effects on memory recall are important when looking at potential factors in depression, which is one of the biggest causes of morbidity (WHO, 2008). Cognitive theories of depression posit that people's thoughts, inferences, attitudes and interpretations and the ways in which they attend to and recall information can increase their risk of depression (Gotlib and Joormann, 2010). The examination of the content of the memories and differences that exist in those with a history of depression or current symptoms might be important in ameliorating future vulnerability. The relevance of designing measurement instruments to measure memory content in the depressed has become increasingly important in treatments aimed at changing unhelpful inferences and is a technique utilised in cognitive and behavioural treatments for depression (Høifødt et al., 2011).

CONCLUSION

That standard techniques have been developed for constructing measurement instruments to add numerical scores has added to the quality and ability to measure attributes of people that are otherwise sometimes difficult to observe directly. The use of these techniques and knowledge of scales does not necessarily provide a good measure, but using such processes gives researchers means of checking on what the measurement instruments purport to measure.

Researchers should have a good knowledge of existing techniques and knowledge of existing instruments that measure similar characteristics of interest. A literature search of relevant or closely related characteristics can help operationalise the concept of interest and is an essential component in terms of judging its quality.

The construction of valid measurement instruments is important to researchers because, ultimately, it impacts practice. By measuring characteristics of interest and converting them into numerical scores, it is possible to gain invaluable feedback on the progress of treatment and its outcomes, which provide indicators and benchmarks for its effectiveness.

FURTHER READING

Chatburn, R. (2011) *Handbook for Health Care Research* (2nd edn). Sudbury, MA: Jones & Bartlett Publications.

Maio, G.R. and Haddock, G.G. (2010) *The Psychology of Attitudes and Attitude Change*. London: Sage.

REFERENCES

Ajzen, I. and Fishbein, M. (1977) 'Attitude–behavior relations: A theoretical analysis and review of empirical research', *Psychological Bulletin*, 84: 888–918.

Beck, J.S. (2011) *Cognitive Behavior Therapy: Basics and beyond* (2nd edn). New York: Guilford Press.

Deeprose, C. and Holmes, E.A. (2010) 'An exploration of prospective imagery: The impact of future events scale', *Behavioural and Cognitive Psychotherapy*, 38b (2): 201–9.

Gotlib, I.H. and Joormann, J. (2010) 'Cognition and depression: Current status and future directions', *Annual Review of Clinical Psychology*, 6: 285–312.

Greene, J. and D'Oliveira, M. (2006) *Learning to Use Statistical Skills in Psychology* (3rd edn). Maidenhead: Open University Press.

Høifødt, R.S., Strøm, C., Kolstrup, N., Eisemann, M. and Waterloo, K. (2011) 'Effectiveness of cognitive behavioural therapy in primary health care: A review', *Family Practice* 28 (5): 489–504.

Likert, R. (1932) 'A technique for the measurement of attitudes', *Archives of Psychology*, 140: 1–55.

Matthews, G., Jones, D. and Chamberlain, A. (1990) 'Refining the measurement of mood: The UWIST Mood Adjective Checklist', *British Journal of Psychology*, 81: 17–24.

Mitchell, A.E.P. (2012) 'The effects of induced negative mood state on recalled autobiographical content and memory'. Unpublished PhD thesis, University of Liverpool.

Osgood, C.E., Suci, G. and Tannenbaum, P. (1957) *The Measurement of Meaning*. Urbana, IL: University of Illinois Press.

Rosenberg, M.J. and Hovland, C.I. (1960) 'Cognitive, affective and behavioural components of attitudes', in M.J. Rosenberg and C.I. Hovland (eds), *Attitude Organization and Change: An analysis of consistency among attitude components*. New Haven, CT: Yale University Press. pp. 1–14.

WHO (2008) *The Global Burden of Disease: 2004 update*. Geneva, Switzerland: WHO Press.

Williams, J.M.G. and Broadbent, K. (1986) 'Autobiographical memory in suicide attempters', *Journal of Abnormal Psychology*, 95: 144–9.

Williams, J.M.G., Barnhofer, T., Crane, C., Herman, D., Raes, F., Watkins, E. and Dalgleish, T. (2007) 'Autobiographical memory specificity and emotional disorder', *Psychological Bulletin*, 133 (1): 122–48.

Debbie Robertson

DEFINITION

'Statistics' are an invaluable means of describing data that have been collected and the making of assumptions based on that data summary (Harris and Taylor, 2008). It is important to know how to interpret basic statistical data and decide whether or not the statistical tests applied are correct (Greenhalgh, 2010), but the availability of easy-to-use tailored software packages to analyse data has meant that many researchers have little understanding of the concepts – statistical and mathematical – behind data handling (Hall, 2008).

Descriptive statistics is a branch of statistics that many people will be familiar with and have used to good effect to *describe* the basic features of the data gathered in a research study to enable readers to interpret them easily. It can be used to provide simple summaries of the outcomes of research. Descriptive statistics, by its very nature, lends itself well, in its various forms, to graphical representation and forms the basis of a large proportion of presented quantitative data analysis.

KEY POINTS

- A basic understanding of the uses of statistics can be helpful in planning and implementing research as well as analysis of any data collected
- Summaries of data allow for the findings of research to be interpreted easily
- Central values – such as mean, median and mode – are commonly used in descriptive statistics
- Standard deviation can give a more accurate representation of values around the central tendencies
- Graphical representation can facilitate the presentation of data to aid understanding

DISCUSSION WITH INTEGRATED CASE STUDY

Summaries of data

Many people, when reading research papers, do not want to be faced with large amounts of raw data. They would struggle to synthesise lots of it into anything meaningful if the data were not summarised by the authors and presented in a fashion that allows the meaning to be clear and unambiguous. Data are often summarised or grouped into the areas of interest or commonality that best describe them (Campbell and Swinscow, 2009).

Sometimes we want to know what 'percentage' of a set of values is one thing or another. Percentages tell us the proportion of time that a particular value occurs. It is a useful way to summarise data when we want to compare the values we are studying with one another. In our case study, a school nurse has been collecting data about smoking in a secondary school population as she wishes to implement a smoking cessation service. She wants this service to be for students aged between 12 and 18.

To justify the need for this service and its roll-out to the students, she conducts a survey of the smoking habits of secondary school children using a representative sample from the relevant year groups in the school. She presents her results to the Board of Governors as part of her justification for the need for the smoking cessation service for the chosen age group.

Data collected by the school nurse in this anonymous survey included age/year group, gender, current smoking status, age first tried a cigarette, numbers of cigarettes smoked daily and desire to cease smoking. The raw data can be seen in Table 32.1.

Table 32.1 Raw data

Current age	Gender	Smoking status	Age first tried a cigarette	Number of cigarettes smoked daily	Desire to cease
12	M	Y	11	5	Y
12	M	Y	10	4	Y
12	F	Y	11	5	Y
12	F	Y	12	5	Y
13	M	Y	12	4	Y
12	F	N	–	–	–
13	M	N	–	–	–
14	F	Y	12	5	N
14	M	Y	11	5	Y
15	M	N	–	–	–
15	F	N	–	–	–
15	F	Y	12	7	Y
14	F	N	–	–	–
16	M	Y	12	8	N
16	M	N	–	.	–
15	M	Y	11	5	Y
16	M	Y	11	10	N
16	M	Y	13	10	N
16	F	N	–	–	–

(Continued)

Table 32.1 (Continued)

Current age	Gender	Smoking status	Age first tried a cigarette	Number of cigarettes smoked daily	Desire to cease
16	M	N	–	–	–
15	F	N	–	–	–
17	F	Y	11	12	Y
17	M	Y	12	14	N
17	M	Y	14	15	Y
17	M	Y	12	15	Y
16	F	N	–	–	–
16	M	N	–	–	–
17	F	N	–	–	–
17	F	N	–	–	–
18	F	N	–	–	–
18	F	Y	13	20	Y
18	F	Y	12	20	N
18	F	N	–	–	–
18	M	Y	15	20	N
17	F	N	–	–	–
18	M	Y	13	15	Y
17	F	N	–	–	–

These data could be summarised better so that when she presents her findings to the Board of Governors, they help to make her case for this service.

She could summarise some of the data by representing them using percentages. The categories of raw values that would be summarised well using this method include gender and smoking status. In the data set, 37 students completed the survey, 18 of them being male and 19 female. To represent these figures as percentages, the calculations would be as follows:

18/37 × 100 = 48.6 per cent were male
19/37 × 100 = 51.4 per cent were female

This represents the basic gender summary of the full data set.

Smoking status is simply given in the raw data as 'yes' or 'no'. Of the 37 students, 20 said 'yes' and 17 said 'no'. To represent these as percentages, we would calculate as follows:

20/37 × 100 = 54 per cent were smokers
17/37 × 100 = 46 per cent were non-smokers

This represents the basic smoking status summary of the full data set.

We can look at these values together to get more of an idea of distribution within the data set by looking at the percentages within each grouping. For example, in the male grouping, there are 18 students. Of those, 13 admitted to being smokers, 5 were non-smokers. In the female grouping, there are 19 students. Of those, 7 admitted to being smokers, with 12 non-smokers.

We can summarise that data, too, as sub-groupings:

13/18 × 100 = 72 per cent of the male grouping smoke
5/18 × 100 = 28 per cent of the male grouping are non-smokers
7/19 × 100 = 37 per cent of the female grouping smoke
12/19 × 100 = 63 per cent of the female grouping are non-smokers

Alternatively, we can summarise them as parts of the whole grouping:

13/37 × 100 = 35 per cent of the group are male smokers
5/37 × 100 = 13.5 per cent of the group are male non-smokers
7/37 × 100 = 19 per cent of the group are female smokers
12/37 × 100 = 32.5 per cent of the group are female non-smokers

These data are more usefully presented this way than in their raw state as they allow comparisons to be made easily between the two groups (male or female, smoker or non-smoker) and their places within the whole group sampled.

Central tendency

The 'central tendency' of a set of data is an estimate of the 'middle areas' of a group of values (Stewart, 2007). There are three main categories of central tendency:

- mean
- median
- mode.

These mathematical terms have specific meanings with regard to statistics.

Mean values

The 'mean' value (or 'average' as it is also known) is probably the most commonly used and well-known way of finding a central value within a group of data.

To calculate the mean value, all the values in a set of data are added up and the total is divided by the number of values within the data set. To take an example from the case study, the school nurse can calculate the mean age of the students by adding all of the ages together and dividing by the number of students in the sample. Adding all the ages together gives a total of 575 and there are 37 students in the sample. The mean age is therefore calculated by dividing 575 by 37, giving an answer of 15.5 years. This value is the mean age of the students in the sample.

Median values

The 'median' value is the number found at the exact middle point of a group of data.

To calculate the median, a simple method is to list all the values in numerical order, then locate the value in the centre of the sample. In our example, there are 37 ages in the list, the exact centre would be value 19 and this would be the median (there are 18 values below it and 18 values above it). To do this, we have to change the order from that listed and rank them numerically from 12 to 18. When we do this, value 19 gives us a median age of 16 years.

The mode

The 'mode' is the value that occurs most frequently within the group of data.

To calculate the mode, the values are listed in numerical order, then each one counted. In our example, we have 37 age values in the data set. The value that occurs most frequently within the data is calculated by adding up how many times each value is represented. This is the mode value and, in this case, it is noted that we have two values occurring most frequently: the ages 16 and 17 both occur 8 times. As there are two modal values, this data set can be described as 'bimodal'.

Dispersion

From our case study example, there are many numbers around the mean, median and mode values. This is not uncommon and is known as 'dispersion'. Most data sets have a dispersal of values, which is why we often calculate central tendencies, to give us an idea of which values have commonality. We can then look at the other values and their distribution around the central tendency, which may also be important to healthcare researchers.

Standard deviation/standard error

The 'standard deviation' gives a more accurate and detailed estimate of dispersion around the central tendency values. This figure shows the relation that set of values has to the mean of the sample (Stewart, 2007).

We know that, in our example, the mean age for when students first tried a cigarette can be calculated. We know that 20 of the students gave an age when they first tried a first cigarette. If we total these ages, we get a figure of 240. To find the mean, 240/20 = 12 years.

The data show that the dispersion around this mean is from 10 to 15 years. We can work out how each value differs from the mean:

10 – 12 = –2 (occurs once)
11 – 12 = –1 (occurs 6 times)
12 – 12 = 0 (occurs 8 times)
13 – 12 = 1 (occurs 3 times)
14 – 12 = 2 (occurs once)
15 – 12 = 3 (occurs once)

Notice that values below the mean have negative differences and values above it have positive ones. Next, we square each difference:

$$(-2)^2 = 4 \times 1 = 4$$
$$(-1)^2 = 1 \times 6 = 6$$
$$(0)^2 = 0 \times 8 = 0$$
$$(1)^2 = 1 \times 3 = 3$$
$$(2)^2 = 4 \times 1 = 4$$
$$(3)^2 = 9 \times 1 = 9$$

Now we sum the values to get a 'sum of squares' (SS). Here, the sum total is 26. Now we divide this by the number of values minus 1 (20 – 1 = 19), so 26/19 = 1.37. This gives us the 'variance'.

To find the standard deviation, we take the square root of the variance, which in this case is 1.17.

Although this may seem complicated, it's actually quite simple. We can describe the standard deviation as the square root of the sum of the squared deviations from the mean, divided by the number of values minus one.

Graphical representation

Many people find data and statistics dry and difficult to interpret, especially if they are presented with large amounts of information. Summarised data can often be made easier to understand by representing them in a graphical way. There are many forms that this can take, including charts, graphs or tables (Freeman et al., 2008). Returning to our case study, the summaries of data regarding the proportions of male and female students and their status as smokers or non-smokers can be easily represented in graphic ways that are very easy to understand (see Figures 32.1 and 32.2).

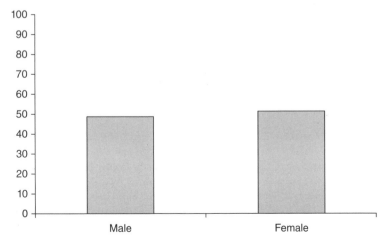

Figure 32.1 Percentages of population by gender

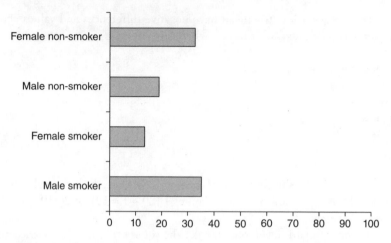

Figure 32.2   Percentages of population by gender and smoking status

CONCLUSION

Descriptive statistics are very useful as they allow us to understand and interpret data that have been collected in the area of healthcare research.

Statistics can be evaluated by non-experts and used to gain a fuller understanding of what to use and when in healthcare research (Greenhalgh, 2010). A basic understanding of simple statistical tests is essential for reading all research. Representing statistics in visual ways, using graphs, bar charts and so on, can also aid understanding by giving a clear visual impact to the data presented.

FURTHER READING

Campbell, M.J. and Swinscow, T.D.V. (2009) *Statistics at Square One* (11th edn). Oxford: Wiley-Blackwell.

Stewart, A. (2007) *Basic Statistics and Epidemiology: A practical guide* (2nd edn). Oxford: Radcliffe Publishing.

REFERENCES

Campbell, M.J. and Swinscow, T.D.V. (2009) *Statistics at Square One* (11th edn). Oxford: Wiley-Blackwell.

Freeman, J.V., Walters, S.J. and Campbell, M.J. (2008) *How to Display Data*. Oxford: Blackwell.

Greenhalgh, T. (2010) *How to Read a Paper* (4th edn). Oxford: Wiley-Blackwell.

Hall, G.M. (2008) *How to Write a Paper* (3rd edn). London: BMJ Group.

Harris, M. and Taylor, G. (2008) *Medical Statistics Made Easy* (2nd edn). Banbury: Scion.

Stewart, A. (2007) *Basic Statistics and Epidemiology: A Practical Guide* (2nd edn). Oxford: Radcliffe.

Mike Morris

There are three kinds of people in the world ... those who can count and those who can't.

(Homer Simpson)

DEFINITION

'Inferential statistics' are usually (but not always) conducted once data have been collected and summarised using descriptive statistics (see Chapter 32). They are used to make inferences (generalisations) from a smaller group of data to possibly a larger one (Salkind, 2004: 9).

KEY POINTS

- Inferential statistics allow researchers to conduct studies on a smaller sample that can be generalised from to apply to the whole of the population from which it was drawn
- Statistical tests provide a p-value, which allows researchers to reach an objective decision as to whether or not to reject the null hypothesis
- Commonly, a p-value equal to or less than 0.05 allows for rejection of the null hypothesis
- Conclusions and recommendations should not be placed on the p-value alone – researchers must also look at the practical/clinical significance as well

DISCUSSION

As populations are typically very large and difficult to access, it is usually impractical, timely and too expensive to investigate an entire population. So, instead, research is usually conducted on a smaller sample (ideally randomly selected) that, hopefully, can be generalised from to apply to the whole of the population from which it was drawn. As researchers usually want to do much more than present descriptive statistics that only relate to their sample, inferential statistical tests are often used as a means of drawing conclusions about a larger population from the results from a given sample.

There are two types of inferential statistics (Powers and Knapp, 2005: 83):

- estimation of population parameters
- testing of hypotheses about population parameters.

The more commonly used of the two procedures by far is the testing of hypotheses.

Estimation of population parameters

This is quite simply the estimation of a parameter, which can be in the form of a mean, a mean difference between two groups (such as placebo versus intervention patients) or a proportion (Polit, 2009: 407).

Subsumed within estimation are 'point estimation', in which the researcher gives a 'best guess' as to the actual value of a parameter based on the calculated value for the corresponding sample statistic, and 'interval estimation', in which a 'confidence interval' provides a range of values having a specified probability that the true parameter will lie within it (Powers and Knapp, 2005).

Testing of hypotheses

Hypotheses (see Chapter 30) are tested using statistical procedures to allow researchers to decide objectively whether the research hypotheses should be accepted or rejected.

If researchers used only descriptive statistics, then it would be impossible to conclude whether or not hypotheses were supported by the results. For example, it was hypothesised that a diabetes workshop improved nurses' diabetes care knowledge. The mean score for the nurses who attended the workshop was 87 out of 100 and the nurses who didn't attend scored 78. From this data alone, it would not be possible to know whether or not the workshop improved their diabetes care knowledge and if the null hypothesis (that there would be no significant difference) could be rejected. This is because, although the mean scores are in the direction that would be expected for the groups tested, it is possible that another sample may have mean scores that are identical, similar or even wider apart. The difference in the mean scores could be explained by chance, such as selection bias (for example, one group including more experienced nurses than the other) or it could in fact be down to an effective diabetes workshop.

Randomly selecting participants to assign to groups should remove issues such as selection bias, but, for researchers to be confident that the intervention was responsible for the difference between the two groups' scores, an appropriate statistical test needs to be conducted to test the null hypothesis. It should be noted that it is the null hypothesis (that the intervention would have no effect) that is tested by the statistical analysis. This is like being innocent until proven guilty – no significant difference must stand until it can be proved otherwise once the data have been collected and statistical analysis performed. One of the most daunting tasks for new researchers is selecting the appropriate statistical analysis from the many that are available.

Selection and interpretation of the statistical analysis

One of the most difficult tasks for researchers is selecting the appropriate statistical analysis to test their null hypothesis. By simply noting a few points about the type of data that has been collected and the research design used, however, it is a relatively straightforward procedure, especially for the more commonly used statistical tests. Presented below is a series of such points, which should guide researchers to select the appropriate analysis for the more commonly used statistical procedures:

- identify the dependent variable (or variables) and assign each to one category of the levels (types) of data (nominal, ordinal, interval or ratio)
- identify whether it is a difference or relationship that is being investigated
- if a difference is being investigated, check whether it is between groups or repeated measures (scores) on the same people – if it is, check how many groups or measures there are.

Once these points have been identified, they can then be applied to simple decision tables (see Tables 33.1 and 33.2). Start by reading the appropriate row for the level (type) of data identified and then the appropriate column for the research design used.

Table 33.1 presents commonly used statistical tests for research designs that have two groups/repeated measures (or scores) or relationships (correlation), Table 33.2 involves more complex research designs, consisting of three or more groups/repeated measures (scores) and studies involving more than one research design (factor). It should be noted that tests conducted in the section labelled 'parametric tests' require the data to be normally distributed and, when testing groups, they are of equal variance (see Coakes, 2012, for more about these procedures).

Once the appropriate statistical test has been identified, the next step is to perform the analysis. Today, sophisticated computer packages drastically simplify the processes that used to involve making calculations by hand. Common software packages used in educational institutions include the Statistical Package for the Social Sciences (SPSS), Minitab and Excel. It is beyond the scope of this chapter to detail all the procedures involved in conducting and interpreting the outputs to all the various statistical analyses, but several excellent texts are available that do (Coakes, 2012; Field, 2013; Pallant, 2010).

The software packages calculate a 'p-value' (significance value). Generally, if this value is equal to or less than 0.05, then you may reject the null hypothesis (Franks and Huck, 1986). This significance value represents the risk associated with not being 100 per cent certain that the difference or relationship observed is down to the hypothesised reason and not to some other unknown reason – that is, there is a 1 in 20 (or 0.05 or 5 per cent) chance the results occurred by chance (Salkind, 2004). So, you can be 95 per cent confident that the results are real and not due to chance. All the emphasis, however, should not be placed on the p-value alone – researchers must look at the practical or clinical significance, whether there is a statistical one or not. Consultation with the descriptive statistics should help with the interpretation, but this also obviously requires researchers to have knowledge in the subject area.

CASE STUDY

A study by Ahuja et al. (2011) investigated glucose levels in the breast milk of obese and overweight mothers. They explored whether glucose and insulin

Table 33.1 Commonly used statistical tests for research involving two groups/repeated measures (scores) and relationships (correlation) (© Mike Morris)

Type of test	Minimum data required	Research designs			Correlation
		Independent groups (between subjects) (two groups)	Repeated measures (within subjects), matched pairs (two sets of scores/ repeated measures)	More than two groups/scores or research designs	
Non-parametric tests	Nominal data	Chi-squared (χ^2) (test for difference)			Chi-squared (χ^2) (test for association)
	Ordinal data	Mann Whitney 'U' test	Wilcoxon signed ranks test	(See Table 33.2)	Spearman's rank correlation coefficient
Parametric tests	Interval or ratio data *plus* data from normal distribution equal variance of samples	Independent t-test (t-test for independent samples)	Paired t-test (t-test for related samples)	(See Table 33.2)	Pearson's product moment

Table 33.2 Commonly used statistical tests involving three or more groups/repeated measures (scores) and more than one research design (© Mike Morris)

Type of test	Minimum data required	Research designs				
		Independent groups (between subjects) (three groups or more)	Repeated measures (within subjects) (three trials/scores or more)	Two (or more) independent groups designs	One independent group design (or more) one repeated measures design (or more)	Two repeated measures designs (or more)
Non-parametric tests	**Nominal data**	Chi-squared (χ^2) (test for difference)				
	Ordinal data	Kruskal Wallis Anova and post hoc analysis	Friedman Anova and post hoc analysis			
Parametric tests	**Interval or ratio data** *plus* data from normal distribution and equal variance of samples	(Simple) one-way independent groups, Anova and post hoc analysis	One-way repeated measures, Anova and post hoc analysis	Two-factor Anova and post hoc analysis	Mixed model Anova and post hoc analysis	Fully repeated measures, Anova and post hoc analysis

concentrations in their breast milk were greater than those of normal weight mothers, which was thought to pose an increased risk of obesity in childhood.

Obviously it would not have been feasible for the researchers to collect data from all lactating mothers classed as normal weight or overweight/obese, so they took a sample of 32 participants with the intention of inferring that the results for this group would be applicable back to the whole of the population from which they were drawn.

A total of 21 non-obese lactating mothers with a pre-pregnancy BMI of between 18.5 and 24.9 kg/m^2 were recruited for Group 1, while 11 overweight and obese lactating mothers with a pre-pregnancy BMI of greater than 25.0 kg/m^2 formed Group 2. Here, the null hypothesis was that, 'There is no significant difference in glucose levels between Groups 1 and 2'.

The descriptive statistics showed the mean (±SD) milk glucose values of the normal weight group to be 32.6±21.8 mg/dL and of the overweight/obese group to be 51.9±20.5 mg/dL. Although the data presented are in the expected direction, this does not allow the researchers to reach an objective decision as to whether to reject the null hypothesis or not. This is where statistical analysis helps researchers, but deciding which one is appropriate is usually one of their most challenging tasks.

The first question researchers should always ask is, 'What is the level of data for the dependent variable?' Here, the dependent variable is the glucose level of the breast milk. This value contains order, distance and origin and, therefore, is classified as ratio data.

The next question to ask is, 'What is the research design?' Here there are two groups (normal versus overweight/obese) and the researcher is looking for a difference.

Bearing these answers in mind, the statistical decision table (Table 33.1) points to the independent t-test as being the appropriate form of analysis. As it resides in the parametric section, there is a requirement for the data to be normally distributed and the groups to have equal variance, which was checked by the researchers prior to beginning the analysis.

The results from the independent t-test revealed a p-value of 0.02. As this is less than the 0.05 significance level, there is a significant difference between the two groups, so the null hypothesis can be rejected.

The descriptive statistics then need to be reviewed to identify the practical/clinical significance of the results. This relies on the researchers' specific subject knowledge. The researchers in this case concluded that, in comparison with normal weight mothers, overweight/obese mothers have significantly higher concentrations of glucose in their breast milk, which could have possible consequences in terms of childhood obesity, although they acknowledged that further studies are required to investigate the underlying mechanisms and consequences this may have (research always generates more research questions!).

CONCLUSION

Inferential statistics are usually an area most students or researchers like to avoid, but they do provide an extremely important tool for reaching an objective decision with respect to rejecting the null hypothesis or not. All inferential statistical procedures provide a p-value. If this value is less than or equal to 0.05, then the null hypothesis can be rejected.

key concepts in nursing and healthcare research

The descriptive and inferential statistics complement each other, providing researchers with all the necessary information on which to base their conclusions and recommendations.

FURTHER READING

Field, A.P. (2013) *Discovering Statistics using IBM SPSS Statistics: And sex and drugs and rock 'n' roll* (4th edn). London: Sage.
Maltby, J., Day, L. and Williams, G. (2007) *Introduction to Statistics for Nurses*. Harlow: Prentice Hall.

REFERENCES

Ahuja, S., Boylan, M., Hart, S.L., Roman-Shriver, C., Spallholz, J.E., Pence, B.C. and Sawyer, B.G. (2011) 'Glucose and insulin levels are increased in obese and overweight mothers' breast-milk', *Food and Nutrition Sciences*, 2: 201–6.
Coakes, S.J. (2012) *SPSS Version 20.0 for Windows: Analysis without anguish*. Australia: John Wiley.
Field, A.P. (2013) *Discovering Statistics using IBM SPSS Statistics: And sex and drugs and rock 'n' roll* (4th edn). London: Sage.
Franks, B.D and Huck, S.W. (1986) 'Why does everyone use the 0.05 significance level?', *Research Quarterly for Exercise and Sport*, 57: 245–9.
Pallant, J. (2010) *SPSS Survival Manual: A step by step guide to data analysis using the SPSS program*. Maidenhead: Open University Press.
Polit, D.F. (2009) *Essentials of Nursing Research, International Edition: Appraising evidence for nursing practise*. Philadelphia, PA: Lippincott Williams & Wilkins.
Powers, B.A. and Knapp, T.R. (2005) *Dictionary of Nursing Theory and Research* (3rd edn). New York: Springer.
Salkind, S.J. (2004) *Statistics for People Who (Think They) Hate Statistics*. London: Sage.

34 Questionnaire Construction

Liane Hayes

DEFINITION

'Questionnaire construction' can be defined as the development of a research tool using a range of questions. These questions can be administered on a form to a large number of people in order to gather data for analysis.

- Questionnaires are self-report tools that are used in nursing and healthcare research in order to generate large volumes of data quickly and efficiently
- Questionnaires may be used to investigate people's attitudes, behaviours, intentions, opinions, beliefs, values, understanding or feelings
- Different types of questions yield different types of data, which can be analysed qualitatively or quantitatively
- Questionnaires should be constructed with a careful eye to their design in order that they will provide the data required to address the research question

DISCUSSION

Questionnaires are used in health sciences in order to gather large amounts of information on a topic. They are developed by generating, constructing, organising, testing and refining questions. Questions are known as 'items' and questionnaires are often referred to as 'scales' or 'measures'.

Scales may measure one thing (in which case they are 'unidimensional') or they may contain several subscales measuring different (though usually related) things (in which case they are 'multidimensional'). Unidimensional tests are considered to be purer than multidimensional ones, though the latter are often used in practice as they tend to be more appropriate. This is because the phenomenon under investigation does not occur in isolation but in the context of other factors (Howitt and Cramer, 2005).

Questionnaires are self-reports of physical or mental phenomena. The use of them in research is described as 'survey research design' (Gravetter and Forzano, 2012). There are many tests already in existence that are often well-established, standardised measures with good levels of reliability, so if a questionnaire already exists to measure the phenomenon you are interested in, you should use that.

Types of questions

Open-ended questions

'Open-ended questions' introduce a topic and allow participants to respond in their own words. While this allows participants the most flexibility in response, it is difficult to summarise or compare responses. This type of data is not suitable for statistical analysis and the usefulness of it often depends on the communication skills and commitment of the participant. Very brief or illegible responses will lack the depth required for any qualitative analysis (Polgar and Thomas, 1995). Open-ended questions are usually followed by a space or a series of lines for the response – the amount of space being left being proportionate to the size of the expected response (Jackson, 2012).

It is often better to avoid using open-ended questions unless there is good reason, as they may be ignored. If you do use them, researchers need to avoid imposing their viewpoint and make sure that the question asks for exactly the information they need (Langdridge, 2004).

Restricted questions

'Restricted questions' limit the response options available to participants. Any number of response options can be offered, as is appropriate to the question. Restricted questions are easy to analyse using frequencies or percentages. They may include an open-ended option, such as 'other', with space to explain or clarify. This style of question is termed 'partially open-ended'.

Rating scale questions

The advantage of using 'rating scale questions' is that they produce numerical data at interval levels that can be analysed statistically (Gravetter and Forzano, 2012). Consequently, rating scale questions are the most commonly used question type in health science research.

Participants are asked to select their response from a number on a scale. Rating scale questions are often called 'Likert scales' (when there are five response points, as in the first such scale developed by Likert in 1932) or 'Likert-type scales' when there are more than five points. There are not usually fewer than five points and not usually more than ten, though there are no rules as to how many should be used.

The assumption is that there are equal spaces between responses, producing data at interval levels. Purist statisticians argue that such data should be analysed at the ordinal level as you cannot say that the differences between the points are the same (Langdridge, 2004; Polgar and Thomas, 1995). In order to avoid this issue, some researchers omit labels from all but the two extreme points ('anchors') on the scale and just leave the numbers. Sometimes the midpoint is also labelled, especially if it represents a neutral response. Not all scales include a midpoint, however. By using an even number of responses, you can force participants to respond in one direction or another (Burns and Grove, 1999).

Participants usually avoid the two points at either end of a rating scale, particularly if they represent attitudes or opinions. This essentially reduces the scale by two points and can lead to a tendency for novice researchers to include more points in their scales. Having too many points, however, can make it difficult for participants to distinguish between them and they will automatically start to group points in their minds – this effectively reduces the scale to something more manageable for them (Gravetter and Forzano, 2012).

If the scale and its labels are the same for every item, participants tend to stick with one response – called a 'response set' or 'yea-saying' (Jackson, 2012). To avoid this, it is better to use a mixture of statements that are either positive or negative in direction to force a change of response patterns in the participants. Where appropriate, you can also change the wording of the point labels to encourage them to make more considered responses.

Structure and design

Questionnaire design should start with searching the literature for the pertinent issues identified in previous research in the area (Bowling, 1997; Priest et al., 1995). If there seems to have been little research published, you could collect information from people who have experience of the area to glean what the key issues are. This could take the form of exploratory interviews or focus groups.

A questionnaire should open with a statement about the focus of the study and why the respondents have been asked to participate. Make sure that there are clear instructions on how participants should complete the questionnaire at the beginning. You may adapt an existing measure for the purposes of the research by, for example, only using certain subscales or altering the wording of questions for a different audience. This is acceptable, but you should report exactly how you have changed it and what effect this has on the reliability and factor structure of the measure.

Only include questions where there is good reason for asking them. Avoid asking speculative questions and only ask questions that are going to be analysable and will help to address your hypothesis. Make sure, too, that the response options given reflect the information you require for your analysis and research question (Rattray and Jones, 2007).

There is an argument for putting demographic questions at the end of a questionnaire because they are considered to be boring and asking them first might put people off or influence how they respond to the rest of the questionnaire (Jackson, 2011). Note, however, that doing so means there is a risk of them being forgotten or left out due to lack of time or loss of interest. The demographic information might be fundamental to the way in which you analyse your data, so if it is not supplied, the data are unusable anyway.

Questions on the same topic and those in the same format should be grouped together to keep the questionnaire simple. You may want the focus of the measure to be obscure, however. If so, avoid grouping questions on that issue, interspersing them throughout the questionnaire.

A questionnaire should be clear and uncluttered and use clear language. Avoid emotionally loaded or leading questions that sway participants in a certain direction. Likewise, 'double-barrelled questions' – that is, the item contains more than one question – should be split into two questions, otherwise it will be too ambiguous to answer (Bowling, 1997). Ask questions about events in chronological order to make it easier for participants to recall and report them accurately (Jackson, 2011).

Questions that are sensitive in nature should go in the middle of a questionnaire as participants are more committed to the research by the time they get to that point and you can ensure you have eased them into these more sensitive questions gently in what precedes them. If a subset of questions has sensitive questions within it, it is wise to put the sensitive questions at the end of that subset and put the whole subset in the middle of the questionnaire (Gravetter and Forzano, 2012).

You might want to include some questions to test for the 'social desirability effect'. If you include the occasional question that is not part of what you are testing for but gives participants the opportunity to present themselves in a 'perfect' light, you then know extreme responses to such questions reflect impossible attitudes and so you should probably disregard the rest of those participants' responses as they will be unrepresentative (Langdridge, 2004).

Number the pages of a questionnaire so that participants complete all of it. Finally, remember to thank the participants for their time and effort and make it clear where the end of the questionnaire is.

Pilot any questionnaire on a small sample of participants, then check that the questions have been completed fully and appropriately. Ask these participants for feedback after they have completed the questionnaire. Such anecdotal feedback may help you to further refine it. You can use item–total correlations, factor analysis or Cronbach's alpha to shorten and refine the questionnaire if you need to (Bowling, 1997; Howitt and Cramer, 2005; Jack and Clarke, 1998; Oppenheim, 1992; Priest et al., 1995).

CASE STUDY

The beliefs about pain control questionnaire (BPCQ) was developed by Skevington (1990). It was informed by the theory of locus of control and two measures of this were considered in the construction of the BPCQ.

Skevington designed 15 items on a 6-point Likert-type scale ranging from 1 (strongly disagree) to 6 (strongly agree). The BPCQ is multidimensional, with items forming three sub-scales – the internal scale (IS), powerful doctors (PD) and chance happenings (CH).

The questionnaire was tested on a range of participants in different states of health and the results compared. Skevington examined the factor structure, reliability, validity and social desirability of the measure. As a result of this analysis, she deleted two of the items (as they weakened the measure) and reworded a third.

CONCLUSION

Questionnaires in nursing and healthcare research can be effective tools to measure several phenomena at once using a large sample. In order for the resultant data to be of good quality, however, care needs to be taken in the design of the measure and the questions it contains. By following established principles of survey research design, it is also possible to investigate psychological issues in healthcare that are difficult to access using other methods.

FURTHER READING

Bowling, A. (1997) *Research Methods in Health: Investigating health and health services.* Maidenhead: Open University Press.

REFERENCES

Bowling, A. (1997) *Research Methods in Health: Investigating health and health services.* Maidenhead: Open University Press.
Burns, N. and Grove, S.K. (1999) *The Practice of Nursing Research Conduct, Critique and Utilization.* Philadelphia, PA: W.B. Saunders & Co..

Gravetter, F.J. and Forzano, L.-A.B. (2012) *Research Methods for the Behavioural Sciences* (4th edn). Belmont, CA: Wadsworth, Cengage Learning.

Howitt, D. and Cramer, D. (2005) *Introduction to Research Methods in Psychology.* Harlow: Pearson.

Jack, B. and Clarke, A. (1998) 'The purpose and use of questionnaires in research', *Professional Nurse,* 14: 176–9.

Jackson, S.L. (2011) *Research Methods: A Modular Approach* (2nd edn). KY: Wadsworth: Cengage Learning.

Jackson, S.L. (2012) *Research Methods and Statistics: A critical thinking approach.* (4th edn). Belmont, CA: Wadsworth, Cengage Learning.

Langdridge, D. (2004) *Introduction to Research Methods and Data Analysis in Psychology.* Harlow: Pearson.

Likert, R.A. (1932) 'A technique for the measurement of attitudes', *Archives of Psychology,* 140: 55.

Oppenheim, A.N. (1992) *Questionnaire Design, Interviewing and Attitude Measurement.* London: Pinter.

Polgar, S. and Thomas, S. (1995) *Introduction to Research in the Health Sciences.* Melbourne: Churchill Livingstone.

Priest, J., McColl, B.A., Thomas, L. and Bond, S. (1995) 'Developing and refining a new measurement tool', *Nurse Researcher,* 2: 69–81.

Rattray, J. and Jones, M.C. (2007) 'Essential elements of questionnaire design and development', *Journal of Clinical Nursing,* 16 (2): 234–43.

Skevington, S.M. (1990) 'A standardised scale to measure beliefs about controlling pain (B.P.C.Q.): A preliminary study', *Psychology and Health,* 4: 221–32.

35 Use of Databases

Nick Syrotiuk

DEFINITION

In the modern world, we are surrounded by databases at every turn. Directly or indirectly, we access information on databases not just every day but every hour. Our university departments, government departments, banks and businesses all rely on databases to deal with important personal and business information.

According to Ullman and Widom (2008), essentially a database is a collection of information that is present over a period of time, often many years. A typical online system today, such as an online banking system, normally consists of a database component and an HTTP web server component.

In the narrower context of academic research, a bibliographic database consists of bibliographic records and/or full-text documents. When researchers conduct literature reviews, they search relevant databases and compile lists of bibliographic citations.

key concepts in nursing and healthcare research

The remainder of this chapter covers the main features of bibliographic databases and the key ones needed to carry out nursing and healthcare research. Unlike other chapters in this book, no case study is offered, other than an exemplar of narrowing and expanding a search. You are prompted to explore some relevant databases in order to discover some of the use you might put these resources to.

KEY POINTS

- Bibliographic databases differ in their scope and style, with most being proprietary, although some have open access
- Databases are searched via an index (list of terms, so careful searching is required to retrieve a manageable number of records)
- Compiling a bibliography is facilitated by reference management software, with the inclusion of a digital object identifier (DOI) being important for identifying a document uniquely

DISCUSSION

The focus in this chapter is solely on bibliographic databases rather than any other kind. The latter include clinical evidence databases, health statistics, directories of all kinds, dictionaries, encyclopaedias, current awareness resources and image collections. Consult Lester (2005) if these kinds of resources are required.

Reitz (2012) defines a bibliographic database in terms of what a database is and the types of information held therein and makes reference to people or groups for whom accessing databases is advantageous:

> A computer file consisting of electronic entries called records, each containing a uniform description of a specific document or bibliographic item, usually retrievable by author, title, subject heading (descriptor), or keyword(s). Some bibliographic databases are general in scope and coverage; others provide access to the literature of a specific discipline or group of disciplines. An increasing number provide the full text of at least a portion of the sources indexed. Most bibliographic databases are proprietary, available by licensing agreement from vendors, or directly from the abstracting and indexing services that create them.

A complex subject requires a long definition and Reitz provides that. Databases are necessarily complex, though it is possible to reduce such complexity into issues of records, indexes, scope, documents and, finally, ownership.

'Databases' are divided into 'files' and files are divided into 'records'. A single bibliographic record in a database describes a single physical container of information called a 'document' (Hagler, 1997). Documents can be textual or non-textual. The most common types of textual documents are books, book chapters, journals, journal articles, conference proceedings, dissertations and government documents. Non-textual documents will not be covered here.

An 'index' is a list of terms you search in order to locate and retrieve records from the database. The most common indexes are author, title, subject, publication date and standard number, usually as an ISBN and ISSN, but there are others. A 'keyword index', for example, can mean one of two things:

- all indexes of the database have been combined into one
- it is an index consisting of every word of every record in the database.

This is an important distinction as the size of the results produced by a search will depend on the format of the keyword index. Indexes and searching are important topics and will be covered in greater detail below.

'Scope' can refer to subject coverage or time period coverage. Reitz specifically refers to subject coverage in her definition above. Thus, a university library catalogue covers all areas of human knowledge whereas the British Nursing Index covers the field of nursing in the UK. Both vary in terms of the time periods covered.

Closely related to scope is the concept of 'bias'. In this context, bias means the publisher of the database chooses to describe and index documents based on national or regional boundaries. For example, Medline has an American bias, whereas Embase has a European one. This is particularly important for healthcare professionals seeking an appropriate system relevant to their work on which to study.

A bibliographic database today may contain a combination of bibliographic records, links to full text documents and the actual full text documents themselves. Even in 2013 not every published textual document is available in electronic form, so be prepared to consult printed materials. It is also common to learn about the existence of an electronic document, but then discover it is only available to subscribers, so be prepared to make an Interlibrary Loan request.

In general, the bibliographic records in a database are owned by an organisation such as a publisher, library, abstracting and indexing service or bibliographic utility, such as Research Libraries UK (RLUK) or Online Computer Library Centre (OCLC). Many databases are 'open access', which means they are freely and openly available to all. Just as many databases are available to subscribers only. Your institution's library will normally subscribe to databases that support the teaching and research at your institution.

The issue of ownership of knowledge is an interesting one, with commercial and philanthropic tensions manifest. It will be interesting to see how far the demands for open access – not just to the public but also to academic researchers – will develop. The pressure from governments to make access to data easier is clear, though knowledge generation and ownership is part of our business and research institutions' core function.

Database search strategy

Bibliographic databases may contain millions of records and it is all too easy to retrieve too many records when searching. It takes practice to develop and refine your search skills.

Generally, start by choosing search terms that are as specific as possible, then widen out your search if necessary. Many systems let you narrow your search by combining search terms from different indexes using Boolean operators (AND, OR, NOT). Sometimes you are allowed to see an ordered list of index terms and can browse through the list (see Figure 35.1).

Note the following from Figure 35.1. The index terms are followed by the number of records in the database containing those terms. This browse list exemplifies the three types of relationships that can exist between terms (Hagler, 1997):

- **equivalence relationships** sets that are similar but different, though have symmetry, are reflexive, separate and transitive
- **associative relationships** things that are alike
- **hierarchical relationships** broader and narrower terms.

One important point is that you can maximise the number of relevant items in your search results by entering the preferred search terms in the search box. In this example, enter 'Cancer Chemoprevention', not 'Cancer Chemoprophylaxis'. (As a rule, omit punctuation from search terms.)

The most important bibliographic databases are called 'union databases'. A union catalogue is simply one large bibliographic database formed by merging a number of smaller databases together. The point of this is that it is then possible to search one union catalogue instead of the other smaller databases separately. Search for books and journal holdings in a union catalogue, but not journal articles. The two most important union catalogues are Copac (http://copac.ac.uk) and OCLC WorldCat (www.worldcat.org or www.oclc.org/worldcat). Copac has a strong UK bias and WorldCat has a strong US bias. WorldCat is particularly useful if you want to know if a publication exists. Both are open access. The bibliographic databases listed in Table 35.1 primarily index journal articles so are better known as journal indexes. These journal indexes are particularly good because they index a large number of high-quality, peer-reviewed journals. Other characteristics of a good journal index include the timeliness of updates, breadth of subject coverage, breadth of time period coverage and an intuitive user interface design. More and more journal indexes now provide abstracts and full text documents, including Europe PubMed Central.

Cancer–Chemoprevention–Popular works	(1)
Cancer–Chemoprevention–Research	(1)
Cancer Chemoprophylaxis	(0)
* See: Cancer–Chemoprevention	
Cancer–Chemotherapy	(300)
* Narrower Term: Cancer–Photochemotherapy	
* See Also: Antineoplastic agents	
Cancer–Chemotherapy	(3)
Cancer–Chemotherapy–Abstracts	(3)
Cancer–Chemotherapy–Bibliography	(3)

Figure 35.1 Example of a browse list resulting from a database search

Table 35.1 Some important journal indexes (in alphabetical order)

Allied and Complementary Medicine Databases
http://www.ebscohost.com/academic/amed

British Nursing Indexhttp://www.proquest.co.uk/en-UK/catalogs/databases/detail/bni.shtml

CAB Abstracts
http://www.ovid.com/webapp/wcs/stores/servlet/ProductDisplay?storeId=13051&catalogId=1315
1&langId=-1&partNumber=Prod-31

Cumulative Index to Nursing and Allied Health Literature, CINAHL Plus
http://www.ebscohost.com/academic/cinahl-plus-with-full-text

Embase/Medline
http://ovidsp.tx.ovid.com/sp-3.8.1a/ovidweb.cgi

Europe PubMed Central
http://europepmc.org

Health Management Information Consortium Database
http://www.ovid.com/webapp/wcs/stores/servlet/ProductDisplay?storeId=13051&catalogId=1315
1&langId=-1&partNumber=Prod-99

King's Fund Library Database
http://kingsfund.koha-ptfs.eu

Maternity and Infant Care Database
http://www.ovid.com/webapp/wcs/stores/servlet/ProductDisplay?storeId=13051&catalogId=1315
1&langId=-1&partNumber=Prod-2694

Psycinfo
http://www.apa.org/pubs/databases/psycinfo/index.aspx

Web of Knowledge
http://wok.mimas.ac.uk

Except for Europe PubMed Central and the King's Fund Database, a subscription is required on the part of the institution you are studying at or your place of work in order to access these databases. Many NHS trusts have licence agreements with their local universities, if access may be permitted there. Web of Knowledge is free to access for students and staff in the UK HE/FE sector.

Compiling a bibliography

While researching any topic, it is important to keep a list of the bibliographic citations for the documents being quoted from or referred to so that they can be included in the bibliography for the study. Nearly every bibliographic database today allows you to download relevant citations to a file. It is common practice to download citations in RIS format and then import them into your favourite reference management software, such as EndNote, a commercial product, or Zotero, a free and open-source software package.

It is important to remember to always include a persistent identifier to a source document in your citations when available. A persistent identifier (or digital object identifier, DOI or doi) is just such a permanent means of identifying a document uniquely. Similarly, an ISBN is to a book as a DOI is to an electronic document. This last identifier is especially important when considering publishing yourself or undertaking higher degree study as often it is a requirement that the references you cite have their DOI as part of the citation.

CONCLUSION

Whether you like it not, consider yourself at home with digital technology or prefer card index systems for information retrieval, databases are ubiquitous in modern healthcare, essential and getting more powerful. Like much of the technology that surrounds us, the work of databases is invisible, gathering swathes of information, collecting and grouping data in our personal and professional lives continuously.

While many of us would not begin to understand how our microwaves heat up the coffee we have left to go cold, we cannot adopt the same blithe ignorance when identifying best practice or evidence for our professional field. As health practitioners, having a rudimentary knowledge of what databases might offer our work, how to perform basic interrogations of them and maintain some systematic approach to our investigations will yield better results than card, pencils and hours in the library.

FURTHER READING

Clamp, C., Gough, S., and Land, L. (2004) *Resources for Nursing Research: An annotated bibliography.* London: Library Association.

Dale, P. (ed.) (2000) *Guide to Libraries and Information Sources in Medicine and Health Care* (3rd edn). London: British Library.

REFERENCES

Hagler, R. (1997) *The Bibliographic Record and Information Technology* (3rd edn). Chicago, IL: American Library Association.

Lester, Ray (ed.) (2005) *The New Walford Guide to Reference Resources: Vol. 1: Science, technology and medicine.* London: Facet.

Reitz, J. (2012) *ODLIS: Online Dictionary for Library and Information Science.* Westport, CT: Libraries Unlimited. Available online at: http://www.abc-clio.com/ODLIS/odlis_A.aspx (accessed 28 May 2013).

Ullman, J.D. and Widom, J. (2008) *A First Course in Database Systems* (3rd edn). Englewood Cliffs, NJ: Prentice Hall.

Part 4

The Research Process

Helen Aveyard with case study by Julie Dulson

DEFINITION

A 'literature review' is a summary of all the relevant evidence that is available on a particular topic. Which parts of it are relevant for inclusion in a literature review is determined by the research question that has been set for the review. The evidence included in a review is usually research evidence, but not always (for example, Katrak et al., 2004).

A literature review can be a prerequisite for an empirical study or a study in its own right. In both cases, researchers search for all the available evidence on the research question. When the literature review is a prerequisite for an empirical study, the researchers aim to identify a knowledge gap and, hence, indicate a need for further study. When a literature review is a study in its own right, the researchers aim to collect all the available evidence in order to develop new insights into the area. Clearly, until a comprehensive search is undertaken it is not always possible to know if there is a gap in the literature, indicating a need for further research or whether there is already a large body of evidence from which new insights can be obtained.

KEY POINTS

- For both types of literature review, the important point is that it should be systematic. Indeed, some reviews are called 'systematic reviews' and these are very detailed, comprehensive reviews, such as those commissioned by the Cochrane and Campbell Collaboration (www.cochrane.org.uk and www.campbellcollaboration.org)
- Other literature reviews do not meet the strict criteria for a 'systematic review' but all should be undertaken systematically and rigorously, to the level of detail that is possible within the constraints of the study
- All researchers and practitioners should be wary of 'reviews' that have *not* been undertaken systematically

DISCUSSION

To ensure that a literature review is comprehensive and systematic, the following four main components are required.

The right research question

Getting the research question right is the first priority when you start your literature review. If your review is a prerequisite for an empirical study, you will have a research question for your overall project, but you may need to adapt or refine it so it is relevant and focused on the literature you need to review to set your study in context. If your review is a research project in its own right, then the question must reflect the focus of your project. For the purposes of this chapter, 'research question' is taken to mean the research question for the review rather than for the a larger study, should the two not be the same.

The research question should be narrow enough to enable you to focus on the detail of the specific area you are researching rather than to be side-tracked, looking at related literature. You will include some background information within your literature review, but should quickly focus down on your specific area of interest.

Many researchers use the PICOT formula to define their research question (Fineout-Overholt and Johnson, 2005; Richardson et al., 1995). This formula assists researchers by ensuring they consider the following elements (spelling out 'PICOT') in their question so that it is balanced yet focused:

- patient or population
- intervention or issue
- comparison or context
- outcome
- time.

An example of a good question using this formula would be, 'What are parents' experiences of caring for a child at home who has complex healthcare needs?' (The P = parents, I = the child with complex healthcare needs, C = in the home, O = parents' experiences, T = nothing as it is not relevant on this occasion.)

If you are doing a literature review as a standalone piece of research, you may find that you refine and alter your research question as your study progresses, depending on the literature you find. This is most likely to be the case if your research project is a component of an undergraduate or postgraduate degree and you have not been given a fixed remit for your research.

The main thing to remember is that the focus of the literature review must fit your literature review question. This might sound simple, but, in reality, it is not uncommon for students to write a literature review that answers a different question from that set.

An appropriate search strategy

Once you have identified your research question, the next task is to search for relevant literature to answer it.

This is an area that has seen big changes in recent years and academic expectations have increased in the light of these developments. With both types of literature review, you are expected to demonstrate that you have undertaken a comprehensive search for relevant literature on your area. It is important to demonstrate that you have not 'cherry picked' what you include in your review.

In order to keep your search as relevant as possible to your research question, write concise inclusion and exclusion criteria for literature that is likely to be relevant and not relevant. These are important as they prevent you from deviating too far from the focus of your research question. It is also useful to consider what type of literature will be most useful to you. This is usually research studies, but you can consider, for example, experiments, qualitative studies and so on. This is referred to as identifying 'your own hierarchy of evidence' (Aveyard, 2010).

You need to access the relevant subject-specific databases and identify which keywords to use for your searches. Remember that the workings of each database are likely to vary and it is important to familiarise yourself with each one in order to use them to their full potential. Keep a record of the keywords and searches you use so that you can give a full account of how you searched for literature when you write up your study.

Despite the increasing use of databases for searching for literature, they are not 100 per cent efficient in identifying relevant literature. That is because it is not possible for those compiling them to identify *all* the potential keywords within every given paper. It is therefore possible that some attributes within papers will not be indexed in a database, so will not be retrieved when a search is conducted using keywords relating to them. For example, a research paper exploring the side effects of a particular drug might discuss three severe side effects and three less severe side effects. Those indexing the paper might index just the three severe side effects. When searching for papers on one of the less severe side effects, this paper would not be identified.

For this reason, it is necessary to have alternative ways to identify relevant literature in addition to searching databases. These might include scrutinising the reference lists of research papers already identified, hand searching physical copies of journals that have published relevant papers and searching for authors who have published on your topic or question.

It is important to keep an accurate record of how and what you have searched for so that those reviewing your work can verify that you have undertaken a comprehensive approach to your review and not left gaps and therefore missed out relevant literature that should have been identified.

Evaluation of the quality of the evidence identified

Once you have identified all the literature that is relevant to your research question, the next stage is to reassess its relevance to your research question and its quality.

To do this, identify the abstracts from your literature search that meet your inclusion criteria and reject those that do not. Next, assess the quality of the literature. There are different ways in which you may proceed. Those undertaking a very detailed, systematic review would assess the relevant papers against strict quality indicators and include only the high-quality studies. This can lead to a very 'select' group of studies for inclusion. For less detailed reviews, you may decide to include less good-quality papers because they nevertheless shed light on your research question, but make sure you acknowledge this fact in your review.

Many researchers use critical appraisal tools to assess the literature they find. These help to ask significant questions of the research papers or other evidence that you have. Remember to access an appraisal tool that is focused on the type of research or other evidence that you are using. There are such tools for discussion papers and guidelines in addition to research methods. The important point is that an appraisal tool does not help you to understand the research; it merely prompts you to ask relevant questions. There is no substitute for thoroughly reading each piece of literature that is relevant to your research question.

Making sense of the literature

The final stage of a literature review is to make sense of all of the relevant papers. For a systematic review, the results of suitable quantitative studies may be combined using a 'meta-analysis', which is a statistical test that gives an overall average of the statistical results of all the papers.

Meta-analysis can only be undertaken if the results of the individual studies can be sensibly combined. When not undertaken, however, there are various ways in which to analyse the literature, such as the also popular 'thematic analysis' (Aveyard, 2010). Thematic analysis involves creating a grid or chart in which are plotted the main results of each paper and then results are compared with each other.

The key to a good literature review

All of the above four components of a literature review should be present, irrespective of whether the review is a prerequisite for an empirical study or a study in itself.

CASE STUDY – JULIE DULSON

This case study relates to my experiences of completing a literature review for my PhD studies. I use the word completing, but that is not accurate as I feel there are always more literature to read, more avenues to explore. My review of the literature so far has enabled me to narrow down my research focus and identify my research question, which has changed several times since I began this process. My PhD studies relate to mental health service users' perceptions of the work of acute inpatient nurses.

At the start of my journey in exploring the literature, I wanted to develop a service user-led assessment tool that would measure qualities of mental health nurses that service users found to be most appropriate for their role. This focus came from my exploration of the literature regarding service users' perceptions of the qualities of good mental health nurses and a desire to measure those qualities in some way. I anticipated a grounded theory approach to developing my assessment tool, but the more literature I read, the more I learned that all service users' perspectives are different – they want to be treated as individuals. I therefore came to understand that developing an assessment tool would be to attempt to create a 'one size fits all' approach, which would be totally incongruent with a service user-led philosophy.

My literature review has enabled me to begin to understand the philosophy and values of my subject area. Developing this understanding has led me to focus on what I was really interested in – service users' perceptions – and identify the appropriate approach to use in my study. I am using an ethnographic approach to my research study, as the more service user literature I read, the more I understand the cultural influences on mental health. This has led me on to explore a wider variety of literature than I included initially – I have read service users' accounts of their experiences on the Internet, for example. While this literature lacks rigour, reading it has enabled me to return to the academic literature, reading it with a fresh pair of eyes, so it has been valuable in this respect.

CONCLUSION

Literature reviews are essential components of empirical studies, but increasingly, are undertaken as studies in and of themselves. Systematic reviews are a good example of this.

For all literature reviews, it is important to conduct them in a rigorous manner so that the literature reviewed is comprehensive.

FURTHER READING

Aveyard, H. (2010) *Doing a Literature Review in Health and Social Care*. Maidenhead: Open University Press.

REFERENCES

Aveyard, H. (2010) *Doing a Literature Review in Health and Social Care*. Maidenhead: Open University Press.
Fineout-Overholt, E. and Johnston, L. (2005) 'Teaching EBP: Asking searchable, answerable clinical questions', *Worldviews on Evidence-Based Nursing*, 2 (3): 157–60.
Katrak, P., Bialocerkowski, A.E., Massy-Westropp, N., Saravana Kumar V.S. and Grimmer, K.A. (2004) 'A systematic review of the content of critical appraisal tools', *BMC Medical Research Methodology*, (4) 22: 1–11.
Richardson, W.S., Wilson, M.C., Nishikawa, J., and Hayward, R.S.A. (1995), 'The well-built clinical question: A key to evidence-based decisions', *ACP Journal Club*, 123: A12–13.

37   Research Design and Method

Annette McIntosh-Scott with case study by
Vicky Ridgway

DEFINITION

The term 'research design' refers to the framework used to guide and inform the research being undertaken, including data collection and analysis (Bryman, 2012; Robson, 2011). As Polit and Hungler (1999) note, the research design drives the fundamental form the research will take and is one of the most important elements in a research study.

The term 'research method' pertains to the chosen means of obtaining and analysing data. Studies may use one predominant technique or employ more than one method (Polit and Hungler, 1999; Robson, 2011).

Both the design and method derive from the overarching research methodology that underpins and informs a research study. This involves the theoretical, political and philosophical contexts within which the research is situated (Robson, 2011).

KEY POINTS

- The research design is constructed taking into account the purpose of the study, its conceptual framework, the research questions, the research methods, the sampling frame and the data-collection procedures
- Designs can be categorised as fixed or flexible, depending on the type of research being undertaken
- Research designs have to be constructed with various constraints in mind and should be achievable within the resources, time and budget available
- Research methods are many and varied, the choice being guided by the focus and aims of the study and which method or methods are best suited to providing the answers or insights sought
- The appropriate research design and choice of the right method or methods are essential to the quality and success of the study

DISCUSSION

A good research design will ensure that there is a logical and clear structure to follow in the operationalisation of the study (Sim and Wright, 2000). Designs can be categorised as 'fixed' or 'flexible' depending on the type of research being undertaken. Robson (2011) states that *fixed* quantitative designs aim to get as much right as possible *before* the major phase of data collection, with pilot work being highly important in this respect, while *flexible* qualitative designs have to get it right by the *end* of the study – hence, are much more flexible. O'Leary (2004) opined that qualitative research should not be done to recipes, but should be fluid and flexible, with strategies developed to answer the research questions. Similarly, Robson (2011) notes that it is common in qualitatively orientated research designs for research aims and questions to evolve and change over time, so researchers should be prepared for such changes.

Although there are different research designs, they do generally have some features in common in their construction. Robson (2011) outlines five key points that each design has to address, which are:

- purpose of the study
- conceptual framework
- research questions or hypotheses
- methods
- sampling procedures.

These are not necessarily set about in a linear way, but all have to be taken into consideration when developing and conducting a research study.

The purpose of the study

This is concerned with ensuring that what the study is trying to achieve is clear – why the research is being undertaken and what the precise focus is. As was seen in the previous chapter, the literature review is often key in relation to this, helping to focus and justify the research and define the purpose of the study.

Sim and Wright (2000) point out that there are two broad purposes of research:

- to test an existing theory – the hypothetico-deductive approach seen in quantitative studies
- theory-building research – the inductive approach seen in qualitative research.

The conceptual framework

Burns and Grove (2009) state that the development of a framework is one of the most crucial, but perhaps one of the most difficult, steps in a research study, noting that the body of knowledge relating to quantitative research is often more defined and developed than that pertaining to qualitative studies.

Essentially, the conceptual framework, or model, can be defined as the interrelated abstractions, models or schema underpinning the study (Polit and Hungler,

1999). Burns and Grove (2009: 146) outline a four-step process for developing a framework, noting that the steps are not necessarily sequential:

- selecting and defining concepts
- developing statements relating the concepts
- expressing the statements in hierarchical fashion
- developing a conceptual map that expresses the framework.

The research questions or hypotheses

A research question defines and clarifies the research and its focus, sets the parameters, gives direction and shape and provides a measure for the success or otherwise of the study (O'Leary, 2004, Robson, 2011).

The characteristics of good research questions are commonly held to be that they are relevant, focused, simple, provide a clear articulation of the research problem or focus, lend direction to the study and can be answered within the resources and time available (O'Leary 2004; Robson 2011). The other important elements to consider in relation to appropriateness are ethical requirements and the practicalities of gaining access. Questions can be framed either as hypotheses or interrogative questions (Atkinson, 2008). Ultimately they are important as they provide the means of choosing the best method or methods for studies.

The methods

As has been seen in previous chapters, there are various research methods that can be used in research. Which one is chosen is guided by the focus of the study and what will be best suited to achieving the aims of the research. The use of mixed methods has become increasingly common, with initial concerns about using methods seen as stemming from two fundamentally incompatible epistemological stances overcome as a result of a willingness to consider research methods as techniques of data collection and analysis that are not wholly entrenched in either ontological *or* epistemological traditions (Bryman, 2012). Indeed, using a combination of methods and triangulating approaches can have considerable benefits, adding a more complete and in-depth view of the areas being researched (Bowling, 2002; Robson, 2011).

The sampling procedures

Deciding on the sampling details involves clarifying who is to be sampled, how they are going to be accessed and what the timescale is. The target population has to be specified, so that it is clear how representative the sample group is and, thus, how limited the findings may be. In quantitative research, power analysis is employed to establish the size of the sample needed to adequately test the hypothesis, while, in qualitative research, there are no criteria for determining sample sizes.

Of equal importance is the choice of the data collection and analysis procedures. Polit and Hungler (1999) note that the selection and development of these, while challenging, are important for the accuracy and robustness of the conclusions.

There should be a high level of compatibility and consistency between the above five characteristics of the design of a piece of research as this will help ensure its quality and success (Robson, 2011; Sim and Wright, 2000). Polit and Hungler (1999) note that the research design also has to specify the measures that will be taken to ensure the integrity and ethical considerations of the study. Sim and Wright (2000) caution that research designs have to be constructed with the constraints and context of the research in mind and are often a compromise between the desirable and the achievable.

CASE STUDY – VICKY RIDGWAY

This case study outlines how I came to select my research design and methods of data collection and how my aims and research questions evolved.

The initial idea for the research came from my own professional experience and developing expertise in the field of nursing older people.

Following a critical review of the literature and policies concerning ageism and attitudes, it became apparent that, although the phenomenon had been researched for a considerable period of time, there were still questions that had not been answered fully and evidence of there still being ageism and negative attitudes towards older people. The available research had predominantly focused on quantitative methods, which perhaps had only offered a snapshot of opinions at a given time and, to me, had not truly answered my initial thoughts and questions.

I therefore started to think how I could research the same phenomenon using a different approach and method. From this, the rationale for the study evolved. It was evident that an enhancement to the field would be to use a new method of data collection over a longer period of time.

So, I proposed that my research design would be a longitudinal study using mixed methods – visual methods, drawings and, to coincide with existing recognised methods and contemporary research in the field, a validated questionnaire. This would enable the gathering of further insights into the phenomenon, to add to the body of knowledge. The longitudinal study element was designed to capture a baseline data set, then monitor and establish alterations to this.

These ideas and consideration of my theoretical perspective led to the development of my research questions and aims. This was the biggest challenge and certainly took longer than anticipated.

Fundamental to the development of the research questions, aims, methods and sample was the need to grasp the research framework. As a result of my own experience, I cannot stress how important this is – to understand what the theoretical basis of the research is, as the whole ethos and approach is developed from these principles. This is something I perhaps had not really appreciated during the development of my emerging ideas. Peers kept asking me what my theoretical perspective was and, initially, I was unclear and stumbled through a description. Then a colleague suggested I reread a text on research foundations, which was enlightening. Clarifying the conceptual framework and theoretical underpinning facilitated the development of the aims and questions, which, in turn, informed the sampling, data collection and analysis.

CONCLUSION

There are many factors that have to be considered when developing a research design and selecting the research methods for a study. The achievability and success of any research endeavour is dependent on getting the design right and selecting the best methods to ensure that the research is robust and all ethical considerations are met.

FURTHER READING

Polit, D. and Hungler, B. (1999) *Nursing Research: Principles and methods* (6th edn). Philadelphia, PA: Lippincot.

REFERENCES

Atkinson, I. (2008) 'Asking research questions', in R. Watson, H. McKenna, S. Cowman and J. Keady, *Nursing Research Designs and Methods*. Edinburgh: Churchill Livingstone Elsevier. pp. 67–73.

Bowling, A. (2002) *Research Methods in Health* (2nd edn). Buckingham: Open University Press.

Bryman, A. (2012) *Social Research Methods* (4th edn). Oxford: Oxford University Press.

Burns, N. and Grove, S.K. (2009) *The Practice of Nursing Research* (6th edn). St Louis, MO: Saunders Elsevier.

O'Leary, Z. (2004) *The Essential Guide to Doing Research*. London: Sage.

Polit, D. and Hungler, B. (1999) *Nursing Research: Principles and methods* (6th edn). Philadelphia, PA: Lippincot.

Robson, C. (2011) *Real World Research* (3rd edn). Oxford: Wiley-Blackwell.

Sim, J. and Wright, C. (2000) *Research in Health Care: Concepts, designs and methods*. Cheltenham: Stanley Thornes.

38   Research Ethics

Martin Johnson

DEFINITION

'Research ethics' are about making sure that the benefits gained from research are as great as possible and any risks are minimised, made acceptable and are freely consented to by participants or their advocates. It is vital that things nurses and other professionals do to patients (interventions) are on a sound scientific footing if at all possible. This means that whether as members of the public or as health professionals, we have a responsibility to encourage research that could improve the patient experience (such as make it safer or more pleasant) whenever we can.

The important point is to be sure that any research does little or no harm. To this end, health authorities and universities have many processes in place that researchers need to follow to gain approval so their research meets high standards and will maximise benefits over any risks.

KEY POINTS

- Autonomy
- Risks and benefits
- Protecting vulnerable people and being inclusive
- Safekeeping of records and data
- Getting ethics approval
- Behaving with integrity

DISCUSSION

Autonomy

Ethics is a branch of philosophy that tries to enable clear thinking about right and wrong in human courses of action. Of course, it is possible for people with different experiences and views to disagree about what might be right and wrong in any situation in healthcare research. For example, early sociological and psychological research into healthcare and human behaviour was often undertaken secretly. This was more or less the norm until a decade or so ago. An example would be a famous study by Rosenhan (1973) in which researchers got themselves admitted to American mental hospitals in order to study the way they were 'diagnosed' and 'treated' by staff even though they did not really have mental illnesses. This study was very influential and made people realise that, often, diagnoses in mental health were not really very objective or consistent. Such a study would be unlikely to be approved by modern ethics committees, however, as the 'covert' approach potentially infringes the assumed right of staff and patients to give consent before being 'studied'. That is, it fails to respect the autonomy of people involved to freely consent or refuse to be studied.

Ethics can involve more than one viewpoint, but autonomy – the right to make our own decisions about things – is very important in all influential perspectives at present, such as those that emphasise human rights and prioritising benefits and risks (Long and Johnson, 2007).

Risks and benefits

Many sources of information about ethics in general and research ethics in particular talk at length about nurses' duties to maintain 'confidentiality' or preserve the 'anonymity' of research participants and organisations. This is a safe initial position to adopt, especially as a student or novice researcher. Even in assignments that only a tutor might read, it is sensible to remove identifiers in references to real people, whether they are to staff or patients. Sometimes, however, and with their consent, these 'rules' can be modified in the participants' interests. For example, some patients give interviews to the press, radio or television about their illness or treatment. Provided they consent and there is no coercion, this can be in everyone's interests as it is important that the public have opportunities like this to learn about modern healthcare.

Risks in research can, of course, be more serious than having one's identity revealed. Some medical procedures and treatments carry a high degree of risk, of side effects or even death. Many cancer treatments, for example, carry high risks because the immune system is severely damaged in order to attack the malignant cells or as a consequence of doing so. This element of risk does not preclude the possibility of the research being undertaken, however, as we would have made little or none of the excellent progress we have in the treatment of many serious conditions, such as breast cancer and some types of leukaemia. In order for such progress to be made, however, many patients will have accepted the risk that, in their particular case, the experimental treatment may not improve their situation, but, in the full knowledge of the facts, they are prepared to accept the risk on behalf of others with their condition, then or in the future.

Although it is a common statement that the 'hospital should do the sick no harm', even the pain of an injection is 'harm'. What we should really say is that, generally speaking, the balance of risks should reduce harm to a minimum for a consequent benefit gained, first for the individual patient and then, perhaps, for wider society.

Protecting vulnerable people and being inclusive

Clearly, although the educational level of adults is very variable, with time spent by staff explaining research, treatments and any risks, most people can make a decision that suits them. Others, however, could be regarded as especially vulnerable in this respect. Young children, people who are temporarily very ill and perhaps in intensive care, some older people who may be losing their mental capacity to make such decisions, perhaps with early dementia, and some other groups of people may need someone to make decisions with or even for them. Age itself, whether people are young or old, is not itself a reason to define someone as vulnerable, so a full assessment needs to be made, drawing on those who knew the person before they became ill if possible.

Indeed, there is a risk that, in being overprotective of individuals or groups like this, we exclude them from research they might possibly benefit from. Clearly, a decision not to study people who are very old or who have dementia, just because they are old or have dementia, would mean such people might never benefit from new treatment or care packages. An excellent paper about this takes the case of people with severe brain injury in a type of coma called 'persistent vegetative state' to make this point (Gelling, 2004). Gelling explains that such people are likely to be excluded from research if we do not think carefully about the balance of minor or absent harms and potentially great benefits. The same applies to many other groups in society, such as people with learning disabilities or whose first language is not English, data from whom are often proportionately less evident than they should be.

Safekeeping of records and data

In healthcare, a good deal of effort has been expended trying to make sure that patient and staff information are kept only for those authorised to read them. Computerisation of information has improved communication of such data greatly in many cases, but it has also increased the risk that such data may become public for the wrong reasons or in the wrong hands. The need to keep data safe has had the negative effect of making such data hard to retrieve, even for legitimate research that may improve the health of patients or the standard of care we are able to provide. There are, however, processes that can allow the proper use of healthcare and patient-related data for research, provided rigorous procedures are followed and, of course, the data need to be stored as securely as current systems allow.

Getting ethics approval

As a result of several cases of poor management of the process of consent and research management (Department of Health (DoH), 2001), getting ethics approval has become much more time-consuming and, arguably, bureaucratic, than it used to be. As noted above, some sociologists saw such processes as irrelevant to their work (Knight and Field, 1981). Today, however, in most cases, research done by staff or students from a university and where data will be collected from the outside world needs, at the very least, to be evaluated by a university or faculty panel that will advise on its suitability. If subjects or respondents are from any kind of health or social care organisation, there are very detailed application processes to follow and these vary from time to time, but your supervisor or tutor can advise you (see also the National Research Ethics Service's website, at: www.nres.nhs.uk).

Behaving with integrity

There is no substitute for integrity. Research ethics approval is often mainly a paper exercise before you do your research, so the detail of what you do at the time may change as you go along and, certainly, the ethics committee will be unlikely to know how exactly you carried out your study.

Good support from tutors or supervisors is important here as they can guide and monitor any study you might be involved in, from a single case study of a patient for an assignment to something much larger, perhaps working with others.

CASE STUDY

Imagine you are worried that members of staff in your unit are not communicating with patients to the extent and in the manner you would like to see and you have read is good practice. You decide that, by saying you are observing and recording the washing of their hands by nurses and all other staff who have physical contact with patients, you can observe their communication skills without them changing their behaviour just for the assessment. We know that, typically, members of staff who know they are being 'assessed' can improve their performance for a few hours, so you decide to observe this behaviour on the pretext of watching something completely different – the handwashing. You believe that in this way you will deflect interest in your real topic, produce more objective data and, thus, the study will be more rigorously 'scientific'.

Think about or discuss with a colleague the following questions about this study.

1. Is 'good science' more important than being completely truthful?
2. Would it solve your dilemma if you got 'consent' for what you were actually looking at afterwards?
3. Have you collected data from patients in a study like this?
4. Given the possible harm (infringed autonomy), are the likely benefits to good practice on your ward sufficient to justify some deception?
5. Might a ploy like this make people less cooperative in the future?
6. Do you think an ethics committee would approve your study if you explained it to them?

CONCLUSION

This is a short introduction to the concept of research ethics. If you are a student, you might work with university or health and social care staff who are doing research as part of their normal work and you are very likely to come across nurses and other health professionals undertaking research in various ways in your practice. Some research is almost invisible. For example, medical staff will already have allocated some patients to different treatments and specialist research staff may collect routine data from them to assess the effectiveness of different treatments. Patients may have agreed to these studies, but often, when very ill, they may feel obliged to try any new treatment available. The nurses' role here can be to explain the research and treatments again and again to patients who may vary in their understanding of what they have agreed to, although nowadays such clinical trials are very tightly controlled by ethics and governance procedures and monitoring.

Other studies, by nurses in particular, may involve you or colleagues in interviews, focus groups or completing questionnaires. Of course, you must decide autonomously whether or not to help with this, but often researchers will teach about their subject or explain their studies in detail, so it's worth considering as a way of learning more about the whole process.

The fundamental question to ask when considering any research question is, 'How much harm can it do?' In nursing research, often the answer is, 'Not that much'.

FURTHER READING

Long, T. and Johnson, M. (eds) (2007) *Research Ethics in the Real World: Issues and solutions for health and social care professionals*. London: Elsevier Churchill Livingstone.
Polit, D. and Beck, C. (2004) *Nursing Research: Principles and methods* (7th edn). Philadelphia, PA: Lippincott Williams & Wilkins.

REFERENCES

DoH (2001) 'The Royal Liverpool children's inquiry report'. London: Stationery Office.
Gelling, L. (2004) 'Researching patients in the vegetative state: Difficulties of studying this patient group', *Nursing Times Research*, 9 (1): 7–17.
Knight, M. and Field, D. (1981) 'A silent conspiracy: Coping with dying cancer patients on an acute surgical ward', *Journal of Advanced Nursing*, 6: 221–9.
Long, T. and Johnson, M. (eds) (2007) *Research Ethics in the Real World: Issues and solutions for health and social care*. London: Elsevier Churchill Livingstone.
Rosenhan, D. (1973) 'On being sane in insane places', *Science*, 179: 250–58.

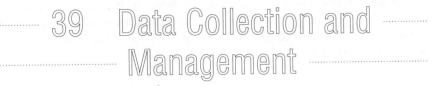

39 Data Collection and Management

Mary Steen

DEFINITION

'Data collection and management' is the information collected by researchers during a study and the steps for monitoring and managing the data.

KEY POINTS

- Data can be collected using both qualitative and quantitative methods
- Researchers are now recognising the value of mixed methods
- Data collection involves some form of observing, assessing, measuring, recording and interpreting
- Data can be collected in a variety of educational, clinical and home settings
- Data can be collected in a number of ways – written, verbally and visually
- Data collected is related to exploring views, experiences, testing out treatments/ interventions or evaluating ways of working

- Data can be 'prospective' (ongoing) or 'retrospective' (looking back)
- Data management involves managing and monitoring collected data
- Data management involves considering how the data will be accessed, stored and disposed of

DISCUSSION

Data collection involves some form of observing, assessing, measuring, recording, analysing, interpreting and reporting. Health-related research can be undertaken in educational, clinical and home settings and the data collected related to exploring views, behaviour, testing out treatments/interventions or evaluating ways of working. The data collected can be 'prospective' – such as exploring patients' views and experiences of the care they are receiving – or 'retrospective' – examining patients' records of care they have received.

Data collection

The type of knowledge that a researcher wants to collect determines the type of research approach, methodology and methods to be used. The overarching consideration when conducting healthcare research, however, is to cause no physical, psychological, emotional or social harm to participants. Here are some examples of what researchers need to consider when undertaking research using different data collection methods:

- researchers, when undertaking interviews, must ensure that the questions are selected carefully and asked in a sensitive manner
- when using observation as a data collection technique, researchers have a responsibility to ensure that participants are informed that they are being observed
- in experimental research, such as a randomised control trial (RCT), the group that are either to receive 'no treatment' or the 'placebo' must consider this option to be acceptable.

Davies (2007) has discussed how it is deemed unethical to not inform people that they are being observed. Researchers must ensure that potential participants understand the concept of what is involved when they consent to taking part in a trial and the fact they may randomly be assigned to a no treatment or placebo group (Smith, 2008).

All this means that researchers need to make good preparations and spend time designing clear and concise information leaflets and provide opportunities to explain in greater detail to potential participants if requested – all of which needs to be planned in prior to and during the recruiting stage of a research study. Informed consent is of paramount importance.

Research governance

It is essential to ensure that research is conducted to a very high standard. 'Research governance' defines how to manage and monitor data collection

(Steen and Roberts, 2011). To this end, in the UK, the Department of Health has published *Research Governance Framework for Health and Social Care* (DoH, 2005). This is a valuable document for health researchers as it outlines the principles of *good* governance that apply to research undertaken within the NHS.

In addition, it is becoming common practice for some institutions and funding bodies to require evidence of a 'data management plan' (DMP) when a research proposal application is submitted. A DMP sets out in clear and concise steps how the data will be accessed, stored, shared, disposed of or preserved if deemed necessary. A plan can include short- and long-term plans for the management of the data. This will depend on the type of data collected, how it is stored – digitally, visually or in written form – ethical and confidentiality issues, as well as institution and healthcare providers' policies and procedures.

The Data Protection Act (1998) is legislation that defines how the processing of data is governed for the protection of personal data in the UK. Local policies and procedures will adhere to the key principles of this act and guide researchers as to the management of research data that will be collected and created. Researchers need to access local policies and familiarise themselves with the necessary requirements. Here are some examples as a guide to the kinds of policies that need to be put in place:

- it is usual practice to store data on a computer that is password protected and to limit access to the researcher alone
- written records of data need to be kept safe and secure, in a locked cabinet, with the personal details of the participants kept separately
- the locked cabinet needs to be in a secure office or room and this should be kept locked when vacant and accessing the office or room could include by means of a secure code system.

Once data analysis has been completed and the results published, then the raw data may be disposed of. Some data may be preserved, however, to support intellectual property rights (IPR).

Data-collection tools and techniques

Data can be collected using both qualitative and quantitative tools and techniques. Which tools will be best to use will depend on the type of research question or hypothesis that has been chosen. Researchers usually choose approaches deemed most suitable for eliciting the kind of data that will answer their research question or hypothesis. Some researchers are now recognising the value of mixed methods to do this and so may choose to use both qualitative and quantitative methods.

Researchers can follow a 'structured', 'semi-structured' or 'unstructured' format, depending on the type of data they want to collect – that is, descriptive, to make an inference, explore meaning or try to understand.

When collecting data

To ensure that the data-collecting process goes smoothly and provides that nec-essary data, first ask the following questions suggested by Steen and Roberts (2011: 740):

- How to collect the data?
- What do I need to know and why?
- What shall I do with it?
- How much time do I have?
- Would another researcher be able to get similar responses?

Data collection for both qualitative and quantitative approaches can appear quite similar, but their application and the retrieval of information differ. Researchers tend to use different data-collection techniques according to the approaches they have chosen.

Some examples of qualitative techniques are observation (participant and non-participant), interviews (face to face, by telephone, online), focus group interviews, examining documents, books, transcripts, digital/visual/media resources, diaries and narratives.

Some examples of quantitative techniques are observation using instruments to measure physiological and biomedical indicators, laboratory experiments, data record sheets, questionnaires and interviews (structured and semi-structured), which may include measurement scales to assess, for example, levels of pain, agree-ment or satisfaction with care.

Qualitative studies

Qualitative research data-collection tools often involve large amounts of written text and this can be gathered from a relatively small number of participants.

Subjectivity is integral when using a qualitative approach as it allows for better understanding by the researcher of the subject under exploration (Robinson, 2002).

Qualitative studies need to be able to demonstrate 'trustworthiness', to ensure that they are deemed to represent the truth. Researchers need to consider the issues of credibility, dependability, confirmability, transferability and authenticity to ensure the truthfulness of qualitative research (Lincoln and Guba, 1985; Polit and Beck, 2008).

Doing this provides a structure to match the key components of the quantitative approach, which are internal validity, reliability, objectivity and external validity.

Quantitative studies

With quantitative research, data-collection techniques are carried out systemati-cally and in a similar fashion, in order to attempt to eliminate bias from the study. Quantitative data can involve measuring how variables interact (cause and effect) and also make comparisons and find correlations. This approach can involve measuring real numbers, such as age or weight, or be assigned to represent people, objects, events, levels of severity, intensity or agreement.

Objectivity is a key element and the data-collection tools used, such as structured questionnaires and structured interviews, are commonly used because they will, as much as possible, collect data objectively. In addition, sampling methods and sample size calculations are used to further promote objectivity.

Quantitative research generates numerical data or data that can be converted into numbers, such as clinical trials or the National Census, which counts people and households.

Questionnaires

Questionnaires are a commonly used data-collection tool in quantitative research, as responses can be structured or semi-structured. They can, however, also be used in qualitative research, but then open questions and/or interviews (with some prompts) are used to allow for the free flow of responses so that respondents' views, thoughts, feelings and experiences can be captured.

The increasing use of computer software programs has influenced how data collection, storage and analysis are undertaken. There is software readily available that can be used to collect both quantitative and qualitative data, such as SPSS and NVivo.

Interviews

The interview is a commonly used technique for collecting qualitative data in healthcare research. A research interview will be carried out to collect data to answer a research question(s) about a phenomenon or topic. The degree of interaction between the interviewee and interviewer can vary depending on the research approach and type of interview. A novice researcher will require some preparation and practice prior to undertaking such an interview.

Interviews can be one-to-one or in a focus group. The options of interviewing by telephone, video conferencing and the Internet are sometimes used, particularly when there are international participants.

Interviews can also be used in quantitative approaches, but would take a different form, such as a survey. A structured format would be used, with predetermined questions asked in a consistent and standardised way with all participants.

CASE STUDIES

A qualitative example

Diaries and interviews are two data-collection tools that give participants opportunities to express their views and experiences. An example would be a phenomenological study that explored midwives' views on confidence when providing intrapartum care. Diaries and semi-structured interviews were used to collect data. The researchers reported that the diaries highlighted data that may not have been uncovered by interview alone (Bedwell et al., 2012).

A quantitative example

Questionnaires work best with standardised, usually closed questions, but some optional 'open-ended' questions can be included to give participants an opportunity to express their personal opinions (Steen and Roberts, 2011). The alleviating perineal trauma (APT) study (Steen and Marchant, 2007) is an example of this method having been put into practice. Its questionnaire recorded responses from women to both closed and open-ended questions during a randomised controlled trial investigating the efficacy of localised cooling treatments for alleviating perineal trauma. The researchers reported that the results indicated cooling treatments can alleviate pain when compared to no localised treatment being given.

CONCLUSION

Data-collection methods are varied and numerous, and which methods are chosen will depend on what will elicit the information needed to answer the hypothesis or research question.

When designing data-collection instruments such as surveys, questionnaires or interview schedules, great care must be taken to avoid ambiguity in the questions or leading respondents. Undertaking a preliminary trial of the instrument is therefore necessary to eliminate errors and design faults.

The quality of the data collected is dependent on the quality and accuracy of the research tools, so whatever ones are chosen should be tested or piloted in order to refine them. On some occasions, the whole research project is undertaken on a small scale first (a pilot study) in order to ascertain whether a full-size version is feasible or not.

FURTHER READING

Bowling, A. and Ebrahim, S. (2008) *Handbook of Health Research Methods: Investigation, measurement and analysis.* Maidenhead: Open University Press.
Griffiths, F. (2009) *Research Methods for Health Care Practice.* London: Sage.

REFERENCES

Bedwell, C., McGowan, L. and Lavender, T. (2012) 'Using diaries to explore midwives' experiences in intrapartum care: An evaluation of the method in a phenomenological study', *Midwifery*, 28 (2): 150–55.
Data Protection Act (1998) (available online at: www.legislation.gov.uk/ukpga/1998/29/contents).
Davies, M.B. (2007) *Doing a Successful Research Project.* Houndmills, Basingstoke: Palgrave Macmillan.
DoH (2005) *Research Governance Framework for Health and Social Care* (2nd edn). London: Stationery Office.
Lincoln, Y.S. and Guba, E.G. (1985) *Naturalistic Inquiry.* Newbury Park, CA: Sage.
Polit, D.F. and Beck, C.T. (2008) *Essentials of Nursing Research: Appraising evidence for nursing practice* (7th edn). Philadelphia, PA: Wolters Kluwer/Lippincott Williams & Wilkins.

Robinson, J.E. (2002) 'Choosing your methods', in M. Tarling and L. Crofts (eds), *The Essential Researcher's Handbook*. Edinburgh: Bailliere Tindall. pp. 64–81.

Smith, G. (2008) 'Experiments', in R. Watson, H. McKenna, S. Cowman and J. Keady (eds), *Nursing Research*. Edinburgh: Churchill Livingstone Elsevier. pp. 189–98.

Steen, M. and Marchant, P. (2007) 'Ice packs and cooling gel pads versus no localised treatment for relief of perineal pain: A randomised controlled trial', *Evidence Based Midwifery Journal*, 5 (1): 16–22.

Steen, M. and Roberts, T. (2011) *The Handbook of Midwifery Research*. Oxford: Wiley-Blackwell.

40   Data Analysis

Elizabeth Harlow

DEFINITION

'Data analysis' is the organisation of raw data into a form that allows the research question to be answered (D'Cruz and Jones, 2004).

KEY POINTS

- Data analysis is central to the research process and planning for the way it will be undertaken occurs from the start of the project
- Although there are numerous approaches to the analysis of data, they can be categorised as either quantitative or qualitative
- Although informed by theory, data analysis is a practical activity that can be less clear cut than textbooks suggest

DISCUSSION

Data analysis influences all aspects of a research project. Consideration has to be given to the analysis of the data when the planning of the project first takes place – when the aims and objectives are established, methodology considered and data are being gathered. Furthermore, for flexible research designs and/or interpretivist methods, additional data might be gathered after the analysis of data collected first of all has begun. In consequence, research might be perceived initially to be a linear process, but, in practice it is often circular, with a repetitious revisiting of aims and objectives, the generation of data and their analysis. The extent to which this occurs is informed by the methodological perspective that is being taken.

In principle, quantitative analysis involves the conversion of raw data, such as observations or recordings, into numbers, while qualitative analysis involves the conversion of similar raw data into words (Denscombe, 2003: 232). In practice, however, there might be occasions when some form of quantification or counting occurs within qualitative analysis – such as when a theme in a text is considered significant due to its repeated occurrence. Similarly, quantitative analysis usually includes an element of interpretation when, for example, it is necessary to judge what 'counts' when phenomena are coded. Nevertheless, understanding analysis as either quantitative or qualitative provides a useful starting point.

'Content analysis' might be either quantitative or qualitative in character and a research project might involve just one or combine both approaches (for example, see Rahill and Mallow, 2011). When used as a quantitative approach, content analysis 'is an approach to the analysis of documents and texts that seeks to quantify content in terms of predetermined categories and in a systematic and replicable manner' (Bryman, 2008: 275).

Content analysis is frequently applied to data that already exist, such as national newspaper articles. So, for instance, a researcher exploring the reporting of nursing and HIV/AIDS in the national press might select an appropriate sample (a range of newspapers over a period of time), then establish a series of questions with which the articles will be interrogated. These questions constitute a coding frame or coding schedule. A coding manual may be written as an aid to answering the questions in a consistent manner (Bryman, 2008: 283). Once the answers have been generated, the frequency with which specific content occurs can be displayed numerically. In its simplest sense, the frequency of articles on nursing and HIV/AIDS can be calculated, but answers to further questions concerning the reporting of the topic might also be gathered – the number of column inches devoted to the topic, for instance (Robson, 2011: 351).

Quantitative content analysis might also be applied to text that has been generated by transcribing the taped recordings of interviews. Berry (2009) illustrates this approach in her research into nurse practitioners' use of clinical preventative services. The interactions between nurse practitioners and their patients were taperecorded and the number of occasions when clinical preventative services were recommended were counted (or quantified). Interestingly, there were fewer recommendations made than researchers had anticipated and fewer than the nurses themselves reported. According to Denscombe (2003: 222), 'The main strength of content analysis is that it provides a means for quantifying the contents of a text, and it does so by using a method that is clear and, in principle, repeatable by other researchers'.

While content analysis is most usually thought of as a quantitative method, as indicated above, there are some researchers who argue that qualitative content analysis is also possible. Drawing on the work of Marlow (2001), D'Cruz and Jones (2004: 153) argue that qualitative content analysis, 'involves the development of codes and categories by the researcher based on theory and literature and their application to documents'. These codes are then deployed in an interpretative analysis of the text – that is, the text is scrutinised for these codes.

While D'Cruz and Jones suggest that qualitative content analysis requires coding categories to be constructed first and then applied to the data, it is also possible to conduct qualitative (or interpretative) analysis without doing this. Instead, the categories or codes are identified from the data themselves.

Robson (2011) – who terms this approach 'thematic coding analysis' – suggests it is a generic approach to the qualitative analysis of data. By reading and rereading the data, codes, which might be understood as theoretical or descriptive ideas (Gibbs, 2007, cited in Robson, 2011: 474), are constructed. An iterative process takes place, by means of which these codes are reconsidered until themes are decided on.

The process of coding depends on whether the themes are to be 'data-driven' or 'theory-driven'. In the former, researchers do not approach the data with prefixed questions, while in the latter the opposite is the case, with the prefixed questions having been generated by means of a literature review. As Robson makes clear, however, both approaches might be used during the same process of analysis. In practice, therefore, a blurring of approaches might take place. Importantly, the codes and themes generated will depend on the aims and objectives of the research. In terms of practicalities, Robson (2011: 482) identifies a number of techniques to generate themes.

Finally, in an attempt to interpret what the 'data are telling you' (Robson 2011: 483), the themes themselves are explored in depth. Quotations are used to illustrate the themes generated and as evidence of the significance they are interpreted as having. As Robson (2011: 486) says, 'Your task is to tell the story of your data in a way which convinces the reader of the merit and trustworthiness of your analysis'.

Thematic coding analysis is closely related to 'grounded theory analysis'. In both of these approaches, the emphasis is on the 'emergence' of the themes from the text. Grounded theory analysis was originated by Barney Glaser and Anselm Strauss (1967) and its 'aim is to *generate* a theory to explain what is central to the data' (Robson, 2011: 489).

The process of analysis involves three specific stages – open coding, axial coding and selective coding. The researchers' engagement with the data is iterative and Pidgeon and Henwood (1996) have referred to this process as the method of constant comparison. Many researchers claim to use grounded theory, but do not comply exactly with the specific procedural techniques, however. In these cases, their approach is more akin to the thematic coding analysis outlined above. Furthermore, the detail of grounded theory has become the focus of debate in recent times as Glaser and Strauss have differed over aspects of its content (Jeon, 2004).

In many instances, computer packages may be used when data are analysed. In terms of content analysis, once the 'rules' for coding have been entered, software packages can quantify documentary or textual content (Robson, 2011: 356). Furthermore, the numerical data generated may be manipulated still further – that is, specific findings can be compared and contrasted. Software packages can also be used for qualitative analysis and applied to a range of research approaches (see Garratt and Klein, 2008, and, for more detail, Robson, 2011: 471). If the sample size is small and the objectives of the project require deep interpretation, however, manual analysis might be still preferred (Hollway and Jefferson, 2000).

CASE STUDY

Although the role of nurse anaesthetist is well established in the USA, this has not been the case in Canada. The recent plan to introduce the role has met with uncertainty among nurses, who have viewed the administration of anaesthetics as a medical rather than caring task.

In response, using the grounded theory approach, Schreiber and MacDonald (2010) established a research project that aimed to 'explore and develop a theory of nurse anaesthesia practice in the USA'. Data were gathered from multiple sources, with the sample of respondents increased over the duration of the project. Fieldwork included attending conferences and visits. A range of observations and conversations were recorded by making notes, while interviews with significant personnel were taperecorded and transcribed. Relevant documents were also collected and analysed.

The researchers achieved the aim of the project and produced a theoretical framework that illustrated the content of the nurse anaesthetist role in the USA. This theory explains the different ways in which the nurse anaesthetists engage with their patients, but also manage the environment of the operating theatre in order that their patients are comforted and protected from anxiety and distress. In the concluding discussion, Schreiber and MacDonald (2010) link these explanations of caring practice to the overarching theories of nursing and what it means to 'nurse'.

CONCLUSION

From the above, it is clear that there are quantitative and qualitative approaches to the analysis of data.

A quantitative content analysis involves applying fixed codes to text and generating numerical findings. In the case study, however, there was an example of the use of grounded theory, in which the researchers did not begin with codes or fixed ideas of any kind, but, by following specified procedural steps, abstracted concepts were allowed to emerge.

In between these two extremes, there are moderated ways in which researchers might approach their task. In short, the examples provided have been arranged along an illustrative continuum.

This brief chapter cannot acknowledge the diversity of research perspectives in this area or the significance of their philosophical underpinnings. Furthermore, in an attempt to make accessible the topic of data analysis, some of the theoretical complexities as well as the messy and uncertain practicalities of the process have been left out. Nevertheless, it is hoped that some of the key elements of what is involved have been captured.

FURTHER READING

Graneheim, U.H. and Lundman, B. (2004) 'Qualitative content analysis in nursing research: Concepts, procedures and measures to achieve trustworthiness', *Nurse Education Today*, 24 (2): 105–12.

REFERENCES

Berry, J.A. (2009) 'Nurse practitioners' use of clinical preventive services', *Journal of the American Academy of Nurse Practitioners*, 21: 454–60.

Bryman, A. (2008) *Social Research Methods* (3rd edn). Oxford: Oxford University Press.

D'Cruz, H. and Jones, M. (2004) *Social Work Research: Ethical and political contexts*. London: Sage.

Denscombe, M. (2003) *The Good Research Guide for Small-scale Research Projects*. Maidenhead: Open University Press.

Garratt, B. and Klein, G. (2008) 'Value of wireless personal digital assistants for practice: Perceptions of advanced practice nurses', *Journal of Clinical Nursing*, 17: 2146–54.

Gibbs, G.R. (2007) *Qualitative Data Analysis*. London: Sage.

Glaser, B. and Strauss, A. (1967) *The Discovery of Grounded Theory*. Chicago, IL: Aldine.

Hollway, W. and Jefferson, T. (2000) *Doing Qualitative Research Differently: Free association, narrative and the interview method*. London: Sage.

Jeon, Y.-H. (2004) 'The application of grounded theory and symbolic interactionism', *Scandinavian Journal of Caring Sciences*, 18: 249–56.

Marlow, C. (2001) *Research Methods for Generalist Social Work* (3rd edn). Belmont, CA: Brooks/Cole.

Pidgeon, N. and Henwood, K. (1996) 'Grounded theory: Practical implementation', in J.T.E. Richardson (ed.), *Handbook of Qualitative Research for Psychology and the Social Sciences*. Leicester: BPS Books.

Rahill, J.G. and Mallow, A. (2011) 'Picuriste/injectionist use amongst Haitan immigrants in Miami-Dade County, Florida: Implications for HIV-related theory', *Journal of Cultural Diversity*, 18 (3): 71–81.

Robson, C. (2011) *Real World Research* (3rd edn). Chichester: Wiley.

Schreiber, R. and MacDonald, M. (2010) 'Keeping vigil over the patient: A grounded theory of nurse anaesthesia practice', *Journal of Advanced Nursing*, 66 (3): 552–61.

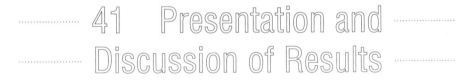

41 Presentation and Discussion of Results

Janice Gidman

DEFINITION

The 'presentation of results' is a very important part of a research report. It is this section that communicates the research findings to the audience, by summarising the analysis of all the data obtained in the study.

The 'discussion' section is where the results are considered in relation to the existing body of knowledge relating to the topic area.

KEY POINTS

- A range of approaches is available to present qualitative and quantitative data
- All tables, graphs and figures must be clearly labelled and explained within the text
- The report should be clear and concise
- The purpose of the report and its audience need to be considered
- Results should be presented and discussed in an accurate and unbiased way
- All claims and conclusions must be justified and any limitations to the study acknowledged

DISCUSSION

This chapter will focus on the presentation and discussion of data obtained from research studies. These are usually written and presented in separate sections, although in some qualitative research reports they may be integrated because of the interpretative nature of the data analysis approach.

The report may be written for a variety of purposes, including undergraduate and postgraduate dissertations, doctoral theses, externally funded research project reports or journal articles. Although the principles are similar, authors need to consider their audience before writing a research report and check the guidelines provided – for example, regarding the level of academic study, author guidelines for a journal or funding body requirements. It is important to remember that, if writing the research report as part of an academic assignment, it is necessary to demonstrate in-depth knowledge of the research process and have the ability to write at the requisite academic level, in addition to communicating the findings of the study.

Presentation of results

One of the main challenges of presenting results is deciding on the best way to communicate large amounts of data within a limited word count. It is important to ensure that these are communicated in an unbiased, informative and interesting manner and the presentation of results is true to the data obtained in the study. There is a range of approaches that can be used to help achieve this, which may differ from each other depending on the methodology adopted for the study. Increasingly, mixed methods are used with health-related research projects and students and researchers therefore need to be familiar with the range of approaches available to enable them to present their results effectively.

Quantitative results

Quantitative research studies often require large volumes of descriptive and/or inferential statistical data to be presented. It is important that, in the report, all the results given are accurate, but it may be difficult for readers to assimilate large amounts of written statistical data. Tables, charts, figures and graphs may be used to summarise data in a visually appealing manner, but these must be accurate and clearly identified and it is necessary to explain and discuss these in the text of the results section. If a hypothesis is stated at the start of the study, then a decision needs to be made as to whether or not it is supported by the data and this decision needs to be justified.

Qualitative results

The presentation of results from qualitative research approaches often comprises themes, narratives, interpretative accounts and direct quotations from respondents. Quotations are often used within the presentation of qualitative results to highlight key issues and engage the interest of readers, but care needs to be taken when selecting exemplars from the data. There may be the temptation to use sensationalist responses that may not be truly reflective of the data overall, but that would lead to bias in the report.

Figures and diagrams are useful ways in which to present the overall conceptualisation of findings in relation to the topic area and these can be visually appealing to the audience.

Discussion section

The discussion section should flow logically from the presentation of results. This is where the findings of the research study are considered in relation to existing literature, theories and policies in the topic area.

In the discussion section, the findings need to be related back to the literature review, to consider to what extent they confirm or refute previous evidence and identify any new knowledge obtained by the research. Researchers also need to refer back to the original research aims and questions and discuss whether or not these have been adequately addressed.

The discussion section should also critically analyse the implications of the research for practice and suggest additional studies to further extend the knowledge base. This should include acknowledgement of the limitations of the study and it is very important that no claims are made that cannot be justified, particularly when reporting small-scale studies.

Writing the results and discussion sections

Reading a variety of research reports is the best way to become familiar with the range of presentation approaches and prepare for writing a research report.

Using critique frameworks to critically appraise the work of other researchers will increase your knowledge and skills and help identify good practice for presenting and discussing the results of research studies using a range of methods. The following lists are suggestions as to specific questions you can use to critically appraise the results and discussion sections. For quantitative reports, ask the following questions (adapted from Coughlan et al., 2007).

- What type of data and statistical analysis was undertaken?
- Was it appropriate?
- How many of the sample participated?

- What is the statistical significance of the findings?
- Are tables, graphs and figures clearly labelled and explained?
- Are the findings linked back to the literature review?
- If a hypothesis was identified, was it supported?
- Are the strengths and limitations of the study, including generalisability, discussed?
- Have recommendations for further research been made?

Here are the suggested questions for qualitative reports (adapted from Ryan et al., 2007)

- Are the findings presented appropriately?
- Are diagrams and figures clearly labelled and explained?
- Have quotations been used in an unbiased manner?
- Has the report been placed in the context of what was already known about the topic?
- Has the original purpose of the study been adequately addressed?
- Are the importance and implications of the findings identified?
- Are the strengths and limitations of the study discussed?
- Are recommendations made to suggest how the research findings can be developed?

When ready to start writing these sections of the research report, you need to formulate your ideas, plan the sections and then write and rewrite it until you are happy that the results are communicated clearly and cohesive arguments have been developed within the discussion. Consider the following case study as an example of how to bring all these elements together.

CASE STUDY

Gidman et al. (2011) undertook a research project to explore nursing students' experiences of support in practice settings. A mixed methods approach was adopted, using self-reported anonymous questionnaires and focus group interviews with students (at the start and end of their programmes) with practice-based mentors.

The data from 272 questionnaires were analysed to produce descriptive statistics. The four focus group interviews were tape recorded and transcribed verbatim to ensure the accurate and unbiased capture of data. This produced extensive amounts of qualitative data, to which thematic analysis was applied and six recurrent themes were identified:

- personal issues
- mentors
- peers and newly qualified nurses
- competence and assessment
- uncertainty of student nurse role
- being part of a team.

The research team had to make important decisions about how to present and discuss these results in the research report and in a subsequent journal article, having to select strategies that ensured they were presented in an unbiased way. A range of graphs, tables and bar charts were used in the full report to provide a visually appealing way of presenting the quantitative data. Due to the word limit set for the journal article, however, it was necessary to summarise these and present them as percentages and rankings.

The extensive qualitative data were presented in themes and key quotations were included to represent the respondents' voices. The research team took great care as to which quotations were selected to ensure that the report was truthful and unbiased.

The discussion section integrated the quantitative and qualitative data and reviewed these in relation to the literature, noting how these were consistent with existing evidence and highlighting areas of new knowledge obtained in this research study. The new areas identified included the additional pressure experienced by students during practice placements; differences in perceptions of support mechanisms between mentors and students; the value of peer support and the priority given to the assessment of competence.

Gidman et al. concluded that support in practice areas is multifaceted and, while acknowledging the limitations of the study in terms of its local context, made recommendations to improve support mechanisms for students. These included the development of peer mentorship systems, a collaborative approach between university and practice placements and a more holistic approach to the assessment of competence.

CONCLUSION

This chapter has considered the purpose and challenges of presenting and discussing results in a research report. This is a vital aspect of the research process and it is important that findings are communicated accurately and effectively. Key to achieving this outcome is the process of determining the purpose and audience of a report and choosing appropriate presentation strategies.

An in-depth understanding of the research process needs to be gained to enable researchers to acknowledge the limitations of their studies and justify any conclusions and recommendations for practice. Remember that, in all stages of the research process – including the presentation and discussion of results – all of the decisions and claims that are made need to be justified.

FURTHER READING

Burns, N. and Grove, S.K. (2009) *The Practice of Nursing Research: Appraisal, synthesis and generation of evidence.* Philadelphia, PA: Saunders. pp. 564–95.

Polit, D.F. and Beck, C.T. (2012) *Nursing Research: Generating and assessing evidence for nursing practice.* Philadelphia, PA: Wolters Kluwer Health/Lippincott Williams & Wilkins.

REFERENCES

Coughlan, M., Cronin. P. and Ryan, F. (2007) 'Step-by-step guide to critiquing research: Part 1: Quantitative research', *British Journal of Nursing*, 16 (11): 658–63.

Gidman, J., McIntosh, A., Melling, K. and Smith, D. (2011) 'Student perceptions of support in practice', *Nurse Education in Practice*, 11 (6): 351–5.

Ryan, F., Coughlan, M. and Cronin. P. (2007) 'Step-by-step guide to critiquing research: Part 2: Qualitative research', *British Journal of Nursing*, 16 (12): 738–44.

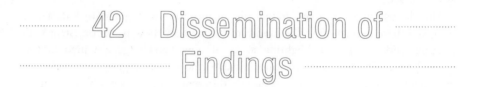

42 Dissemination of Findings

Elizabeth Mason-Whitehead and Michael Hellenbach
with case study by Mike Brownsell

DEFINITION

Dissemination of research and research findings is a crucial stage in any study and means to 'spread the word' about the valuable work that is going to be or has been conducted, including envisaged or actual outcomes. By publishing the results of their studies, researchers broaden the existing body of knowledge and contribute to the continuing discussions in their fields, as well as promoting change and improvements in practices and procedures.

During the dissemination process, researchers engage with stakeholders, fellow academics and people who may have contributed to, or participated in, the study. By doing so, they can help bring different interest groups together and facilitate communication between them.

Researchers will usually be asked to provide a detailed dissemination plan when applying for ethical approval for their investigative projects. In this context, how and to whom the outcomes of a study will be made accessible should be strategically planned to maximise the potential impact of the study. Consequently, scientists need to identify their audiences and the means by which they will reach them.

Dissemination, however, is not confined to publishing research findings, but applies to every stage of the research process and informing others about progressing investigations does not necessarily have to be one-dimensional. As a result of presenting or publishing updates about their work, researchers may obtain useful

key concepts in nursing and healthcare research

and critical feedback, helping them to broaden their own views and avoid problems or difficulties in their projects.

As will be explained in greater detail below, research and research findings can be disseminated by a range of different means and activities, such as publications in newspapers, journals or books, presentations during meetings and conferences with practitioners and academics, but also while teaching students or professionals.

KEY POINTS

- Research findings must be reported honestly
- Irrespective of the size of the study, a professional report will follow a plan (see Table 42.1)
- The data must support the analysis, discussion, conclusions and recommendations
- The report content should be written in a way that is cognisant of the target audience
- A shorter summary can be very helpful for large studies and provide the lay members of the fundholding organisation with a comprehensive overview
- It is important that time is taken to write and review the report thoroughly, checking findings, grammar, spelling and references. Your name and that of your institution will be attached to the report, which will be circulated widely!
- Acknowledge all the contributors to the report
- You may need to have your report printed professionally, so ensure that you have included this in your budget and timeframe
- Deliver your report on time. This is good professional practice and you may be looked on favourably for future work

DISCUSSION

The dissemination of findings is crucially important. Indeed, Bowling (2009: 180) argues that, 'Investigators have a moral duty to ensure that their results are disseminated to the target audience'. Unless there is a prerequisite to present the findings, however – for example, if the study is being funded – this final stage of the research process may not be given the focus and attention it deserves. The reason for this is not clear, but it may be that the exhausted researcher is just tired and fed-up!

This chapter provides an overview of the dissemination process, including influences on dissemination, structure of dissemination and types of dissemination.

Influences on dissemination

As researchers, novice or experienced, how and why we disseminate what we have learned is not always considered as clearly or logically as it might be. In the following extract from a systematic review of dissemination frameworks, Wilson et al. (2010: 12) identify the breadth and complexities of disseminating research findings, saying it is:

a planned process that involves consideration of target audiences and the settings in which research findings are to be received and, where appropriate, communicating and interacting with wider policy and health service audiences in ways that will facilitate research uptake in decision-making processes and practice.

Frameworks for dissemination

Employing a framework can give a structure and focus to dissemination that we otherwise would not have had. A number of dissemination frameworks are used (Wilson et al., 2010) by researchers, although many do not use such techniques. In Table 42.1, there are five points to consider when planning disseminating your results.

Structure of dissemination

Dissemination of research findings follows a recognised structure, informing readers as to how the research was undertaken, as shown in Table 4.2.

Table 42.1 A framework for dissemination (adapted from McGuire, 2001)

Questions to be addressed for dissemination	Researchers' response
What is your institution or organisation?	The institution where you are based and conducting your research
What message do you want to communicate to your audience(s)?	The message you convey will depend on your audience(s) and whether they are, for example, professionals requiring a detailed breakdown of results and/or an overview of findings for a lay audience
How are you going to communicate your research findings?	You can communicate your findings in a variety of forms, including reports, conferences, publications and the media
Who are the audience(s)?	Knowing your audience(s) is crucially important as you will present your findings accordingly (see second question)
Who are your findings going to be communicated to?	The institution receiving your findings. This is likely to be your fundholder, but it may include other interested bodies such as charities and user groups

Table 42.2 A structure for dissemination of research findings

Title, author/s
Acknowledgements and fundholders
Short summary, Abstract
Aims and objectives/research hypothesis (if appropriate)
Research methods and design, including ethical approval, data set, measurements, process of data analysis
Findings and analysis, discussion, limitations, conclusions, recommendations references, appendices

Types of dissemination

The main types of dissemination, choosing how to use them and the formats they can take are summarised in Table 42.3.

As can be seen, dissemination of your research findings can take a number of forms, which are discussed below.

Reports

Reports vary considerably from a simple overview of a project to a thorough account and detailed analysis of each finding. This will be reflected in the word count required.

It is customary to submit a number of hard copies of a report (approximately three) and follow this up with an e-mail attachment. If the research has been funded, you will normally know at the start of the project the type of report the funding body requires. Interim reports are sometimes requested, so the funding body can be assured that money is being spent in accordance with what has been agreed, progress is being made and deadlines are being kept.

Table 42.3 Types of dissemination

Type of dissemination	Choice of dissemination	Format
Report	Fundholders require a final report. Sometimes an interim report is requested	Printed paper report(s) and electronic submission
Writing for publication	Journal publications are an excellent way to disseminate findings to academic and professional colleagues	Journal papers for professional and impact factor journals
Conference presentations	Appropriate conferences may provide many opportunities to disseminate research via oral presentations and posters, as well as forming new collaborations with conference attendees	Core and theme papers usually require a 20–30-minute PowerPoint presentation followed by 10 minutes for audience questions. Posters are usually an A1-size sheet presenting the study in a condensed form
Professional meetings	In many organisations, including hospitals, there are regular meetings where new research that has been conducted by their employees is presented	Professional meetings, talks to lay groups, presentations to fundholders and informal discussions
Media	The media may hear of your research, find your subject interesting and ask you to be interviewed by a journalist. If you wish your study to reach a wide audience, the media can be very useful	Interviews with local or national radio, television, newspapers or magazines

Mohammed has recently completed his first research project and submitted his report to the local charity funding his project. The charity's director has written to Mohammed, complimenting him on his final report, which she said was clear and concise. It was also noted that Mohammed had written a very 'user-friendly' short summary that the laypeople involved in the charity found easy to understand. Additionally, the health professionals involved in the charity were impressed by how the recommendations were supported by his data analysis.

Mohammed was pleased with this response and attributes the success of his report to gaining experience in one of the school of health sciences research teams before he won his first bid and became principal investigator of his own research study.

Writing for publication

Being published in healthcare research is concerned with making research findings known to an audience that may consist of professional colleagues, laypeople or both. The most likely types of publications will be journals or books. Journals fall into two main categories: professional and impact factor journals.

Professional journals

These journals may be sponsored by a professional organisation and have a wide readership. Some can be bought at newsagents. They are usually peer reviewed, but the review process is generally shorter than for impact factor journals and the contributions are frequently professional articles.

This type of journal could be a good choice where research findings have a strong application to practice and be of national significance rather than global appeal.

Impact factor journals

Contributions to impact factor journals can be significant on a number of levels. The 'impact' of the category name refers to the number of citations of articles published in that journal.

Impact journals cover a wide range of subjects and methodologies. Deciding which one to submit your paper to can be confusing, so, if you are new to publishing, you may be wise to take advice from your tutor or supervisor. The papers submitted to such journals can take a number of forms, which one you select will also depend on the message you want to convey and which one is most suitable for the work you want to publish.

Generally, the editors of impact factor journal are looking for original contributions that will make a contribution to the literature. Research papers are the submissions most often received. If yours is chosen, it is your opportunity to disseminate your research study in a paper of approximately 3000–5000 words. Once published, you may receive feedback and discussion from readers and other interested groups who may wish to collaborate with you on future projects, invite you to present at a conference or, more rarely, but it does happen, to help fund further research projects related to your study.

Books and book chapters

Disseminating your research in the form of a chapter in an edited book or as a book in its own right is not common, but it happens. More likely, you may use your research study as an example of a research methodology within a chapter. For instance, you may be writing a chapter on qualitative research and present one of your studies as an example of interviewing vulnerable groups and the challenges this poses for the researcher.

CASE STUDY

Alana has completed her research assignment and identified two possible ways of publishing it with her tutor, Jane – namely, a literature review paper and the findings from her study on the evaluation of a patient's new menu. The literature review paper will present a review of papers relating to hospital food, critically examining cultural differences, initiatives and interventions and how other countries have approached the challenges of hospital meals. Jane has advised her that this paper should be submitted to an impact factor journal, reminding Alana of the scarcity of high-quality literature review papers. They have identified a hospital management journal and Alana is using her literature review chapter as the framework for this paper.

Alana and Jane have reviewed her evaluation study carefully and concluded that it is rooted in professional practice. Jane is mindful that Alana's study involved only one UK research site with a small data set and has a practical rather than a theoretical application. For these reasons, they decided to submit Alana's paper to a professional and national journal, as its readership consists of clinical colleagues.

Jane and Alana reflected on the decisions they had made and discussed the importance of understanding the role of journals in academic and clinical practice. Alana commented that she was not aware that there was such a large number of journals or, indeed, the differences in their approaches. Jane advised Alana that, now she has just completed her research journey, she is about to commence another – that of writing and submitting a paper.

Over the next few weeks, Jane and Alana met to discuss and review the progress of Alana's submissions. Alana began with the literature review paper. She read the author guidelines carefully and set out the headings for her paper as instructed. The substance of her paper was taken from her literature review chapter and this was incorporated into the new piece. Jane updated her review and changed the format accordingly. She found Jane's advice of reading other literature reviews – particularly those from her chosen journal – very helpful as she wrote her own.

Alana asked her friend and fellow student, Debski, to read and give feedback on her paper, which she found very helpful. Jane informed Alana that submitting a paper can be a rather daunting prospect, so she advised Alana to read the instructions carefully and attach each file as requested. Alana found this a lengthy and frustrating process, but she did successfully complete all the information and upload her files, in the end commenting that it was a rewarding experience. With new confidence, Alana submitted her second paper and Jane's assistance was not required.

The editors from both papers returned the reviewers' comments and both articles required amendments. Alana, while being disheartened by this, was soon reassured by Jane, who was pleased to see that the amendments were minor. Jane encouraged Alana to respond to the reviewer's comments within the next few days, which she did. Both papers have now been accepted for publication and Alana feels immense satisfaction, knowing that her study has been disseminated widely to her academic and clinical colleagues.

Conference presentations

Presenting at conferences has a long history as an arena in which professionals from all backgrounds can present their findings. During conferences there are opportunities to share similar and differing experiences relating to professional interests.

There are several questions to consider before submitting an abstract to a conference panel to review, including the following:

- What are your funding sources and do they cover the cost of the conference and your accommodation?
- Who is your audience and is it relevant to your research study?
- Your experience and confidence are important – is this is your first conference?

If you are in doubt or it will be your first conference, seek advice from your tutor or supervisor and talk with people who have presented at conferences. For a first time, you may want to start at a local or national level rather than embark on an international one.

When submitting your abstract, you will be invited to select a format you would like to give your presentation in, which will be an oral paper or a poster presentation. There are three types of oral papers:

- **core paper** – you will be asked to present for about 30 minutes and set the scene for the theme papers
- **theme paper** – approximately 20 minutes long, with 10 minutes for questions
- **symposia paper** – a number of contributors present their work, which is good for joint collaborations and new presenters as there's safety in numbers!

Poster presentations are an ideal way to begin your conference experience, as an alternative to presenting. They provide an opportunity to become familiar with what conference settings are like and the ambience. You will be asked to set up your poster at the beginning of the conference and then meet and talk with the people who view your poster. You may also be asked to give a brief talk as you stand next to your poster. This combination of poster and oral presentation is becoming increasingly popular.

The submission guidelines will inform you of the conference's submission deadline and when the inclusion decisions have been made regarding which papers and posters have been accepted.

CASE STUDY – MIKE BROWNSELL

Having spent 18 months developing a Web-based standardised numeracy assessment tool (SNAP), the collaboration team were keen to share both the tool and their experiences with the wider academic community. As with many collaborative projects, however, deciding on how and where to disseminate the knowledge gained proved as challenging as developing the actual tool.

There was more than simply a numeracy tool to share and differing potential audiences that might find what we had to say interesting from a range of perspectives. Should we aim for an information technology conference to present and discuss the development and software design processes and the human interface challenges encountered? Would it be better to introduce the tool to a pedagogically focused audience to discuss the eLearning methodology and educational model behind the learning resource component? Alternatively, should we aim for a conference exploring policy development and change management to present how new stakeholders, late to the original collaboration, subtly altered the original aims and how the resulting mission creep was managed? Finally, should we start by presenting regionally, nationally or be brave and try for an international conference and go for maximum exposure?

Fortunately, past experience had proven that the conference we chose to submit our abstract to would have to be academically sound, with abstracts being blind peer reviewed and a previous reputation for successful event organisation. This pointed towards the larger national or international conferences. A review of database search engines using keywords such as 'elearning' conference, 'Healthcare AND education' conference and 'Health AND Education AND Policy Conference' soon gave us a shortlist of likely conferences. As might be expected, many proved to be international conferences.

Being a financially shrewd project manager, I had sufficient project funds to part support several of the key collaborators so that they could attend and jointly present a paper at the *Nurse Education Today* and *Nurse Education in Practice* (NETNEP) 2012 conference in Baltimore. The reasons for choosing this particular conference were that it reaches a wide audience of the largest professional group using the tool and, being sponsored by two of the most popular nurse education journals, it had multiple breakaway workshops covering all the aspects considered earlier and, finally, the quality of other presentations we would be fortunate enough to see while at the conference was peer review assured and likely to lead to the full publication of our own paper in a special edition of the journal later in the year.

Meetings

Meetings are an intrinsic part of professional life and, some would argue, many are not as productive or valuable as they claim to be. Meetings and committees that include a relevant presentation are generally welcomed, particularly if the audience is to receive new knowledge.

Researchers may be asked to present their findings to a professional meeting or a meeting of laypeople. The dissemination of research findings to both of these groups is an important component in the research process. Understanding the target audience(s) is critical and ensuring that sensitive and sometimes unwelcome findings are presented appropriately is essential.

CASE STUDY

Two student midwives, Amanda and Tiger Lily, have been invited by the hospital women's health research group to present their research findings to their monthly meeting. Both students became quite well known within the hospital for securing funding from their professional body to carry out a research study that has now been reported in the local press. The research project was based on an intervention where the students intensively visited travelling families based in the area, which included pregnant women.

Amanda and Tiger Lily have little experience of attending professional meetings, let alone giving a presentation. They conveyed their anxieties to Dr Singh, the chair of the group. He reassured them that they would have an interested and friendly audience. He also suggested that they tell their story of their interest in antenatal women from travelling communities, how they secured their funding and worked their way through each stage of the research process, as well as how their recommendations are linked to their research findings.

Amanda and Tiger Lily became very apprehensive when they heard that Rachael Goldstein, a senior representative from their awarding body, was to attend. Dr Singh reassured them that this was normal practice for fundholders – to not only to see how their money was being spent but also to be informed about their progress. The meeting was just as Dr Singh predicted, with a flurry of enthusiastic questions from professional colleagues, including Rachael.

Amanda and Tiger Lilly were subsequently asked by the travelling families to discuss their research. The students hired a nearby hall. They wanted to create a friendly atmosphere, so they served refreshments and placed the chairs in a semi-circle. Their talk was informal and informative, heightened by their new confidence. The travelling families asked many questions and offered their views on the intervention.

When the student midwives reflected on their experiences, they felt that Dr Singh's support had been invaluable. Amanda and Tiger Lily had followed his advice, prepared their talk and did not try to be anything other than what they are – two young midwives, showing promise for the future.

Media

The media is becoming increasingly important as a way of disseminating research findings, particularly if a subject appeals to the general public. There is a wide range of media, including newspapers, television, radio and the Internet.

While it can be a great opportunity to discuss your findings on the 'airwaves' and be interviewed by journalists, it is advisable to not approach or respond to the media without first gaining permission to do so from your institution. Its press office will usually work in collaboration with you.

CASE STUDY

Lucy and Vimay have evaluated a breakfast club study undertaken in a local secondary school. If the breakfast club is shown to be a success, then future funding will be provided.

Sarah, a journalist working for the local newspaper, approached Lucy and Vimay requesting an interview. The two researchers worked in conjunction with the school and their university, giving Sarah a comprehensive interview and providing her with all the correct facts about their study. The piece Sarah wrote included information from the headmistress of the school, who was able to confirm to the local newspaper that funding for the next three years is secure for students to have breakfast prior to their lessons.

Reflecting on their experiences, Lucy and Vimay said that they found their research study to have been worthwhile, but they were cognisant of working with their institution and their fundholders.

CONCLUSION

Ultimately, healthcare research is about developing our knowledge in order to enhance the quality of people's lives. If we do not disseminate our research effectively, we do not further our knowledge, develop our ideas and theories and the groups of people we have researched will receive no benefit from our work. We therefore have to be able to convey our research results in an honest, coherent and clear manner.

This chapter has emphasised that however we disseminate our research findings, whether it be orally or in writing, we have a duty to ensure that our means of presentation is appropriate for our target audience. As healthcare researchers, we have an obligation to inform the public of our findings and a personal and collective responsibility to those people we have researched. They may be vulnerable or belong to minority groups and to them we have an additional responsibility: we could be their 'voice' and it is imperative that they are heard.

The efforts we make in disseminating our findings, whether by the written or spoken word, or both, are worthwhile because they could contribute to new policy, be an agent for change and make a difference.

FURTHER READING

Aveyard, H. (2009) *A Beginner's Guide to Evidence Based Practice in Health and Social Care.* Maidenhead: Open University Press, McGraw-Hill.

Polit, D.F. and Beck, T.C. (2008) *Nursing Research: Generating and assessing evidence for nursing practice.* Philadelphia, PA: Lippincott Williams & Wilkins.

REFERENCES

Bowling, A. (2009) *Research Methods in Health* (3rd edn). Maidenhead: Open University Press, McGraw-Hill.

McGuire, W.J. (2001) 'Input and output variables currently promising for constructing persuasive communications', in R. Rice and C. Atkin, *Public Communication Campaigns* (3rd edn). Thousand Oaks, CA: Sage. pp. 22–48.

Wilson, P.M., Petticrew, M., Calnan, M.W. and Nazareth, I. (2010) 'Disseminating research findings: What should researchers do?: A systematic scoping review of conceptual frameworks', *Implementation Science,* 5: 91 (available online at: . www.implementationscience.com/content/5/1/91).